Felon
FITNESS

How to Get a
HARD BODY
Without Doing Hard Time

**TREY TEUFEL, NASM Certified Trainer
& WILLIAM S. KROGER, Attorney at Law**

▲adamsmedia

Avon, Massachusetts

Published by
Adams Media, a division of F+W Media, Inc.
57 Littlefield Street, Avon, MA 02322. U.S.A.
www.adamsmedia.com

ISBN 10: 1-4405-2659-1
ISBN 13: 978-1-4405-2659-6
eISBN 10: 1-4405-2746-6
eISBN 13: 978-1-4405-2746-3

Printed in the United States of America.

10 9 8 7 6 5 4 3 2 1

Library of Congress Cataloging-in-Publication Data
is available from the publisher.

The information in this book should not be used for diagnosing or treating any health problem. Not all diet and exercise plans suit everyone. You should always consult a trained medical professional before starting a diet, taking any form of medication, or embarking on any fitness or weight-training program. The author and publisher disclaim any liability arising directly or indirectly from the use of this book.

Many of the designations used by manufacturers and sellers to distinguish their product are claimed as trademarks. Where those designations appear in this book and Adams Media was aware of a trademark claim, the designations have been printed with initial capital letters.

Interior exercise photos by William S. Kroger.
Photos on pages x, 8, 126, 136, and 198 © istockphoto.com/francisblack,
dundanim, PerlAlexander, leezsnow, coolmilo.

This book is available at quantity discounts for bulk purchases.
For information, please call 1-800-289-0963.

Dedication

To my wife, Jill, and my daughters, Willow and Olivia, for sharing their love and happiness. And, for sharing their morning workouts and stretches with me.

—William

To Dr. Lee Teufel, PhD, my mom and dad, Michael Latimer for his guidance, Emily G., Sunil Malhotra and Sumi Pendakur, Mark Smith, Larry Ames, Frank Zito and Elevation Fitness, Jessica Porter, Ned Haspel, Richard Cardona, Jason Pease, Barbara Miletich, Linda Wallem, Lara Ingraham, Keith Knopf, Equinox, Body360 Nutritionals, APLA/T2EA, Rusty and Stephen, Lynn, Transcendence Theatre, and my clients for their support during the writing of this book: C. Peters, Dr. Parviz Javdan, John Solberg, Randall Gitter, Sam Loyola, Chelsey Santry, Kevin Kassover, the Mashians, Farid Pakravan, Jeff Jampol, the Milkens, and the Sandlers.

—Trey

Acknowledgments

We would like to thank our main men on the inside, Shant Der Boghossian and J. Pinedo. Through their insights we were able to fully grasp the inner workings of the prison system and the workouts necessary to help them maintain their sanity and save their lives. We would also like to thank all the inmates who allowed us to publish their workouts: Dennis James Baltierra, Jeffrey W. Goldstein, Israel Alberto Guillén, Tom McDonald, Manuel Meza, Alejandro Perez, and Anthony Sarmiento (also RJ Kaushaul and Yu Li for their insights into the federal prison system and allowing us to visit and eat chicken wings and strawberry cheesecake with them).

And a special thanks to our agent, Bob Silverstein of Quicksilver Books Literary Agency, and our editors, Brendan O'Neill and Katie Corcoran Lytle of Adams Media, without whose support this book would never have been a possibility.

Contents

Foreword

When Bill and Trey approached me about writing the foreword to this book, I didn't give it a second thought. Anyone who is passionate about health and fitness will tell you that helping those who want to improve their well-being is very gratifying.

I landed in California State Prison in 1996, and within months of my arrival the weights were being loaded onto bulldozers and taken away from us prisoners. I was out of shape and now faced an arduous task of getting fit. Or so I thought.

Many people believe that it is impossible to get big or gain muscle without the use of free weights. Well, that is far from the truth. Granted, without weights you won't get huge. But with proper training, diet, and rest you can get in great shape and look good at the same time. Back then, I knew nothing about strength, endurance, or explosive training, let alone building size and power with the use of my own body weight. But, because I was around hundreds of inmates every day, it was easy for me to network and gather many different weight-free exercises—and it didn't even take as much time as you may think.

It is a common belief that prisoners are in such good shape because we spend hours working out. From what I see every day and from my own experience, forty-five minutes to an hour a day four to five times a week is all anyone needs to get in excellent shape. Couple that with determination and consistency and you'll be on your way to a better you in no time.

Whether you are looking to build muscle, burn fat, or just try something new, within the pages of this book you will find workouts that not only are challenging but will put you on the path to reaching your ultimate goal—a healthy body and a strong mind.

—J. Pinedo, K-14865

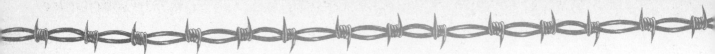

Introduction

In the mid-1990s, the California Department of Corrections and Rehabilitation removed weights from all of their prison yards and left inmates to create their own exercise programs based on body-weight exercises. The result? Fit and healthy inmates who have learned to use their bodies as functional pieces of equipment with exercises like squats, pull-ups, and push-ups to build their stamina, burn off excess body fat, and increase their strength.

Being in shape is a matter of life or death for these inmates. Either they are fit enough to fend off an attack or they could end up in the morgue. It's that simple. But your life depends on you being fit as well. You likely don't have to worry about being attacked by a gang member with a makeshift knife, but you do have to be concerned about both staying healthy and improving your health. Fortunately, you can achieve a hard body without doing hard time and building up muscle and endurance isn't as time intensive—or as expensive—as you may think.

You may be thinking: "Of course inmates are in incredible shape! They don't have anything to do *but* exercise." Inmates do have a lot of free time, but they're only allowed to use a small portion of that time to exercise. In fact, most of the felon-approved workouts that we share with you here take less than sixty minutes to complete. And, since these workouts can be done anywhere from a prison cell to the privacy of your own home, the time you save by not driving to the gym will be well spent.

But perhaps more importantly, you'll learn without a shadow of a doubt that the only piece of equipment you need to get in shape is your body itself. No shakes. No supplements. No gym fees. No home equipment. No magazines telling you how easy it is to get fit (it has never been easy, nor will it ever be easy). No personal trainers. No fancy clothes. No smoothies. No pills. No energy drinks that make you jittery and send your heart beating out of your chest. All you need is you—and some objects that you likely have lying around your house already.

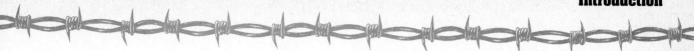

You don't even have to be physically fit to get started on this program. When we first started asking inmates about their fitness routines some of the men told us that they lacked strength when they were first incarcerated, and others couldn't run a quarter of a mile when they first started serving their time. But little by little they found themselves getting stronger and running faster, and the well-balanced inmate workout plans you'll find here will help you do the same. However, these workout plans will benefit different people in different ways: If you're already muscle-bound, you'll learn how to improve your range of motion with exercises like butterflies and cherry pickers. If you're already an aerobic bad-ass, you'll learn how to increase your strength with push-ups, squats, lunges, and prison dumbbell exercises. And if you're just starting out, you'll find combinations of aerobic routines and weight-training exercises to help you dodge a bullet or pry a shank from the hand of a fellow inmate—even if, in reality, that bullet is just a toy thrown by your three-year-old and the shank is a wallet you're trying to pry out of the mouth of your golden retriever. You'll also find tips that tell you how to enhance your personal workout program and help you eliminate exercises from that routine that often lead to injury.

So read on to find out what the inmates have to share about their personal routines, learn how to stretch properly, find an exercise philosophy that's right for you, and start working out—with conviction.

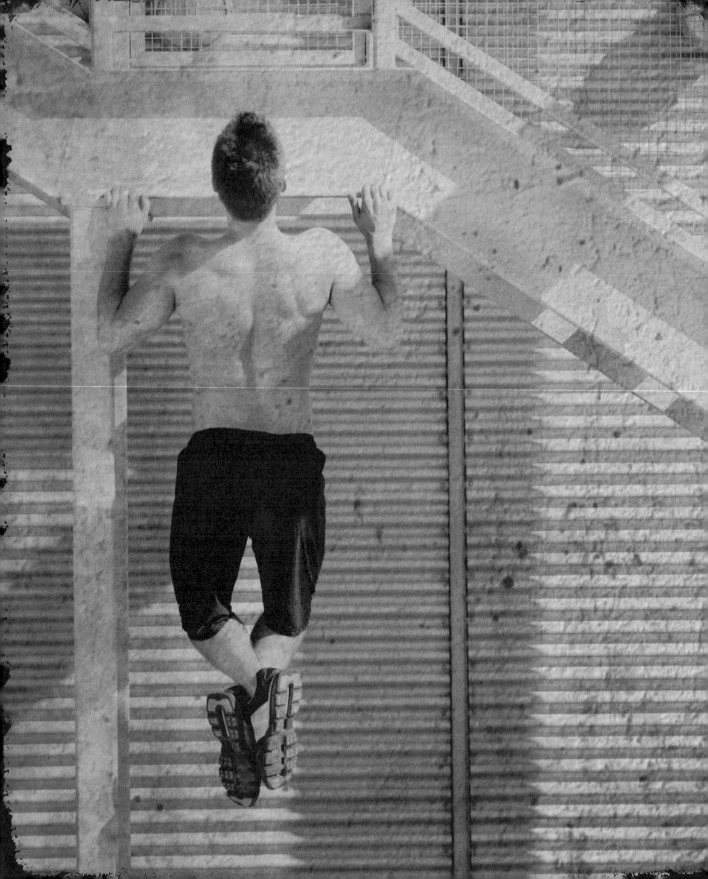

PART 1

Prison Dumbbells and At-Home Ingenuity

While the majority of the exercises and workout routines that you'll find throughout the book require nothing more than your own body weight, occasionally you will need to use some equipment. We're not talking about expensive free weights or an exercise machine that will sit in the corner of your basement for years, though. If an inmate doesn't have access to these materials, you don't need to use them either. Instead, look around your house and you'll find that you probably already have everything that you need. You just need to learn how to turn these everyday items into workout gold.

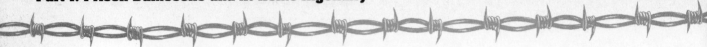

Prison Dumbbell

Many of the exercises you'll find in *Felon Fitness* require a simple form of resistance. You can add that resistance to your workout by using a "prison dumbbell," a homemade weight consisting of magazines tied together by strips of bed sheets and secured with tape. Believe it or not, you can make your own prison dumbbell with little effort. All you need are the following:

- ✖ Magazines
- ✖ Heavy-duty tape
- ✖ A set of bed sheets
- ✖ Scissors
- ✖ A scale (if you want to be precise with the weight of the dumbbell)

You'll use this homemade weight for curls, flys, front raises, lateral raises, lawn mowers, upright rows, kick-outs, hammer curls, overhead presses, bent-over rows, and more. To make a prison dumbbell follow the directions on the next page:

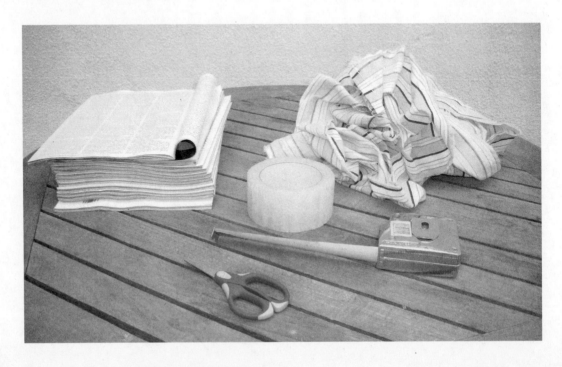

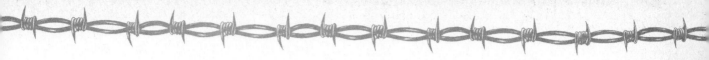

1. Once you have your materials ready, start by ripping the bed sheets into five equal strips, each 2 to 3 inches in width and at least 30 inches in length. Note: If you're having trouble ripping your bed sheets, scissors will certainly come in handy; they're hard to come by in prison, but feel free to make an exception.

2. Next, stack your magazines on top of each other evenly. Twelve magazines of equal size will weigh approximately 10 pounds, and a stack of forty magazines will weigh between 30 and 35 pounds. You can easily adjust the weight of your dumbbell by adding or subtracting the number of magazines to suit your current level of strength/conditioning.

3. Tie one strip of your ripped sheet around the center of the stack of magazines. Tie the strip as tight as possible. Then tie a second strip on the left of the dumbbell, and a third on the right side. Make sure all three strips are tightened evenly. If not, your dumbbell will be uneven, which may cause unbalanced muscle growth and possible injury.

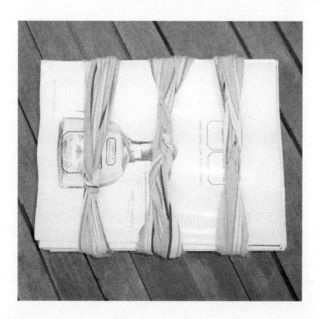

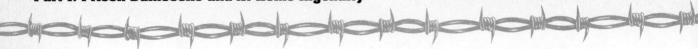

4. Next, tie a fourth sheet strip to the sides of your stack of magazines to secure the paper in position.

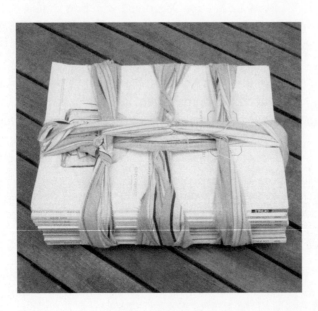

5. To finish up you need to create a handle for your dumbbell. To do so, roll up a magazine into a firm bar about 1½ inches in diameter. Once the magazine is rolled up you can either tie a shoestring in the middle of it or just tape the magazine so it doesn't unravel. The handle you just rolled up will have a small hole at the end of both sides like a telescope. Insert your fifth sheet strip through that hole, tie it around the stack of magazines, then secure with tape, and check for areas that might be loose. Any wobbly sections should be addressed with more tape or additional sheet strips.

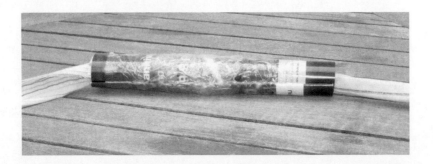

Once you've finished constructing your prison dumbbell, it should look like the following:

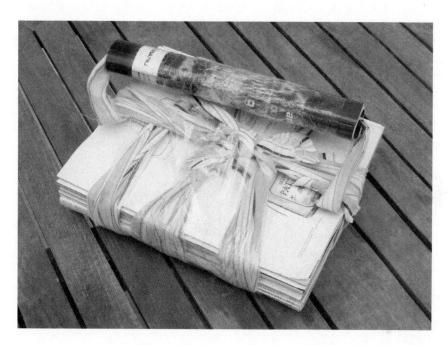

WORDS FROM THE YARD:
MANUEL MEZA, H-37966

A prison dumbbell consists of about forty magazines (*GQ*, *Stuff*, *King*, *Latina*) [that] are all close in size, with good weight to them. Legal paperwork, transcripts, Case Law of at least 15 inches thick, combined with the forty magazines will give you about 50 pounds or so.

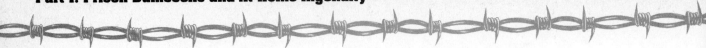

You can and will use different grips for different exercises while incorporating the prison dumbbell. Shoulder raises, upright rows, bent over rows, and reverse curls use an overhand grip. Curls and concentration curls use an underhand grip. Experiment with how you hold the dumbbell and use what feels most comfortable for you.

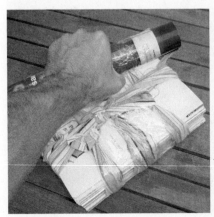
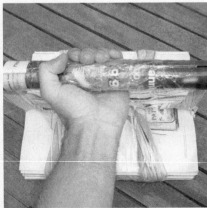

overhand grip   **underhand grip**

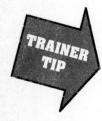

TRAINER
TIP

If you don't want to make your own prison dumbbell, you can also buy weights that suit your fitness level. Start by trying out three pairs of dumbbells (15 pounds, 20 pounds, and 25 pounds, for example). If you use them consistently and feel you're strong enough, purchase heavier weights, but keep the ones you have in case you need them down the line.

At-Home Ingenuity

The prisoners use their creativity to make dumbbells out of magazines and bed sheets, but since you have more items at your disposal you can be even more creative. If you don't have magazines handy, use buckets of water to double as your gym equipment. Just measure the weight of the bucket on your bathroom scale and you're good to go. If you don't

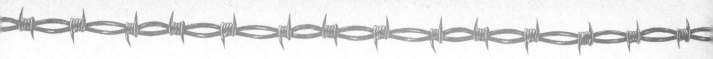

have buckets, gallon milk jugs or soup cans are a great size for shoulder, biceps, and triceps exercises. You can also use phone books if you're looking for something hefty. And if you're doing curls you can attach something (cans of paint, for example) to a broom for extra weight.

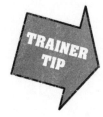

We recommend the use of actual dumbbells if you need to lift weights that are precisely calibrated to weight amounts that are exact to the pound. Working out with magazines will have the same effect as lifting iron dumbbells, but actual iron dumbbells will be a bit more consistent in terms of their mass.

Besides dumbbells, other kinds of gym equipment can be improvised from household items. For example, if you can't do push-ups from a horizontal position, place your hands on something higher than the ground—a bench, the seat of a chair, the back of your couch, a coffee table, or the back bumper of your car. These will aid your chest and leg work during diamond push-ups, wide-grip push-ups, plyometric push-ups, bench dips, Bulgarian/Romanian squats, step-ups, and more. Doing back exercises is tricky, but you can compensate by using exposed beams or strong pipes for pull-ups. If you have kids, you can even do pull-ups on their swing set.

There are many options out there that we haven't discussed here, but use your imagination and feel free to be inventive—our inmates certainly are.

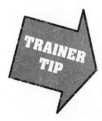

Enjoy exercise outside during the spring, summer, and early fall. The sunshine will boost levels of vitamin D, improve your mood, and keep you from colliding with objects in your home.

PART 2
Exercises

In this section you'll find a variety of exercises for each body part that inmates really do on the inside. Keeping your workout routine varied and exciting with these different exercises will prevent injury, boredom, and plateaus. Definitely repeat the exercises you enjoy, but also challenge yourself with exercises you don't particularly like. People often stay away from the exercises that are most difficult for them, highlighting where they are weakest. Instead of accepting defeat, make your weakness your strength by attacking the exercises you hate. For example, if you are great at push-ups but can't do a squat with good form, don't get stuck in a push-up rut. Stay on your feet and address your issues with the squat, and you'll thank yourself when you begin to see progress.

While performing these exercises, it is of the upmost importance that you maintain good form to avoid injury. Quality over quantity is a mantra to repeat while doing any of these exercises. Measure your success with the progress you make in the number of repetitions you can do as opposed to the amount of weight you can lift. That shift in how you see the value in your workout is one you'll learn to love.

CHAPTER 1

Back

Inmates understand that someone with a solid back is a person you don't want to mess with. Strong back muscles, the second largest muscle group in your body, can help pull an attacker off a friend or cellmate, climb a wall or fence while escaping an assault, or simply pick up a loved one during a scheduled visitation. But a strong back will serve you well in everyday movements too. The muscles that make up the back are responsible for many aspects of such movements including standing, holding your shoulders back for good posture, picking items up from the ground, and any and all pulling actions. You may think that these everyday movements are things that you just do, but, in fact, they're a very unconscious aspect of physicality that need to be addressed actively, consciously, and much more often. Much of the population is hunched over computers, smartphones, and other electronic devices and, instead of just accepting slouched posture and sore backs, we all need to think even more about how we sit and stand and make a special effort to strengthen these sometimes overlooked muscles. To make sure your back is strong try the exercises in this chapter.

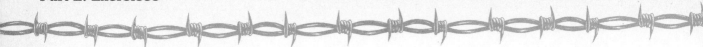

Pull-Ups

Perhaps the most tried-and-true exercise for developing back strength is the pull-up. If you're looking to develop your *Latissimus dorsi* muscles (commonly called "lats"), which are located on the side of the back below your shoulders, and enhance your "V" shape so your shoulders and back remain wider than your waist, look no further than this exercise.

To do a normal pull-up, grab a bar, a beam, or anything sturdy and, with your feet off the ground, pull your body up until your chin is higher than your hands. Lower yourself with a slow and controlled motion before repeating. A pull-up with good form (as shown in the images below) has the head up, the chest out, and the shoulder blades pressed down.

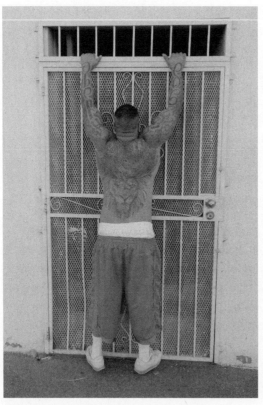 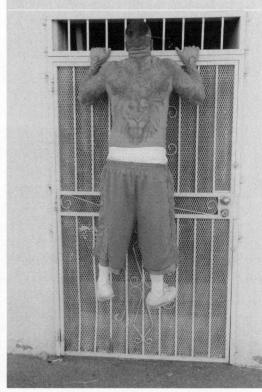

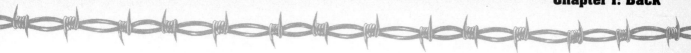

Where to Do Them

Use any solid beam or supported bar/rod to add pull-ups to your workout. If your budget doesn't allow for one of the countless brands of pull-up bars sold in sporting goods stores, use a pull-up bar in a park, as shown in the images below, or use a tree branch. If you want to get really hard-core like they do in prison, just flip your bed up on its end and do pull-ups on the frame.

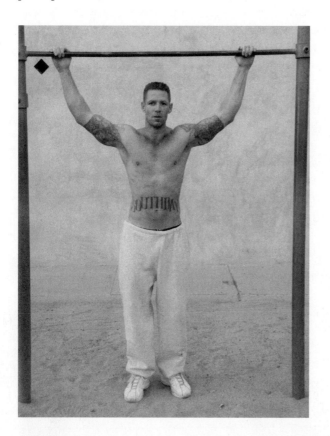

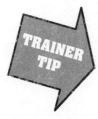

TRAINER TIP

Exhale when you exert. Simply put, breathe out when you perform the lifting portion of any exercise.

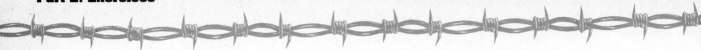

Pull-Up Grips

As with the prison dumbbell discussed in Part 1, you can use different grips when you do pull-ups. Along with mixing things up and keeping you from getting bored, using these different grips utilizes different muscles so that others may rest. For example, if you complete workouts with underhand grip pull-ups for a month before switching to overhand pull-ups, you'll notice that when you return to underhand pull-ups a couple of weeks later that you can do more repetitions with greater ease because you've given the muscles responsible a break. It's important to perform new variations of pull-ups (and all other exercises for that matter) to avoid performance plateaus.

UNDERHAND GRIPS

If you're a pull-up beginner, an underhand grip makes the movement easier. This grip forces the biceps to do even more work than they're used to. You likely already have strong biceps from lifting and carrying countless items, so the underhand pull-up gives you the opportunity to develop back strength. That strength in turn will aid you in turning your grip over for the more difficult overhand pull-ups.

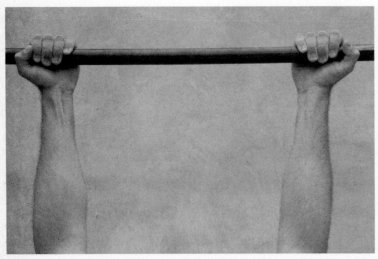
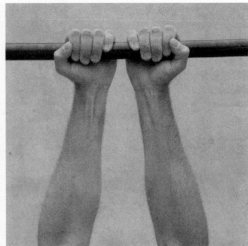

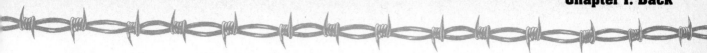

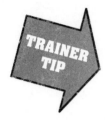

If you work out with a partner, try friendly contests to see how many repetitions you both can perform for any exercise. That spirit of competition will motivate the "loser" to try harder to improve his or her number of reps, while the "winner" will work hard to stay ahead.

OVERHAND GRIPS

An overhand grip keeps the biceps in the game, but forces your back to do the bulk of the work. Overhand grips make pull-ups harder to perform because they require greater use of the "little lats," the small muscles above the lats and under the shoulder on your back, as well as the lats. Chances are that you'll experience more soreness in the back part of your armpit after doing overhand pull-ups.

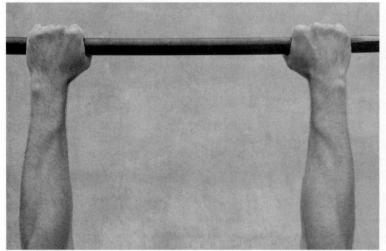

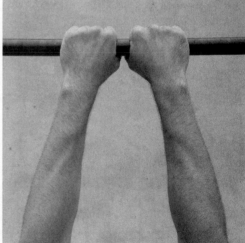

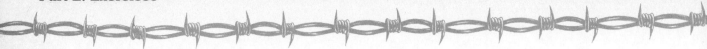

ALTERNATED GRIPS

Alternated-grip pull-ups, where one hand grips overhand while the other grips underhand, are a great way to mix things up in order to avoid plateaus in results. This unusual exercise is also more realistic for your everyday life. After all, pulling yourself up from any surface is rarely done with an even grip, so why train for such instances during your workouts?

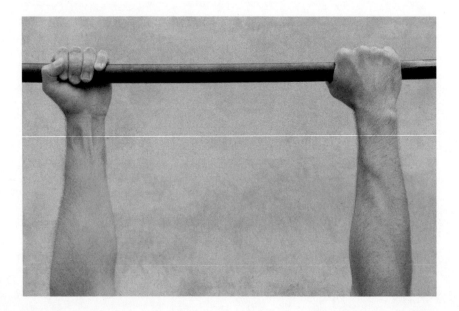

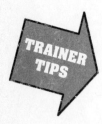

* Always work to keep your shoulder blades pushed down. You can avoid a lot of shoulder issues by being strict with your form.

* Enhance any pull-up variation by holding your knees up throughout the entire movement. That knee-hold will allow your abs to be more engaged and will help make the pull-up that much more challenging.

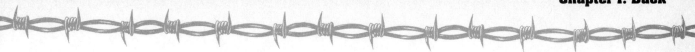

What If I Can't Do a Single Pull-Up?

Developing the level of strength necessary to do a pull-up can be a challenge. Remember to start with underhand grip pull-ups to get your lats going before you transition to overhand varieties. If that is still too hard, do what is known as a "negative" pull-up: Jump up into the end position (with your chin higher than the bar) and slowly lower your body down. Once your arms are completely straight, jump up and repeat. Try three sets of 8 to 12 pull-ups if you want to get bigger and stronger. If you're looking for a leaner look and want to tone, do 15 or more for each set. Keep in mind that fewer reps induce muscle growth and strength, whereas more reps burn more energy and lead to greater endurance but less growth.

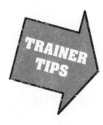

* Be patient. Losing weight, developing strength, and gaining lean muscle mass takes time. Consistency is the key to achieving all three.

* Wear gloves or use some other form of protection while doing pull-ups to avoid tearing up your hands.

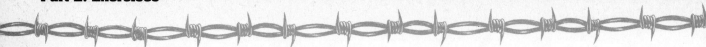

Chain Breakers

Work the muscles that hold your shoulders back for good posture by performing Chain Breakers. With your arms straight out in front of you at shoulder height, pull your arms back while bending at the elbow, simultaneously squeezing the middle of your back and opening/stretching your chest. Pulse your arms back three times to make it a "three-count Chain Breaker."

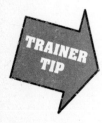

TRAINER TIP

Pretend like you're elbowing somebody when doing Chain Breakers. Imagine you're at a bar and want to get rid of the person who's annoying you. Throw those elbows back sharply!

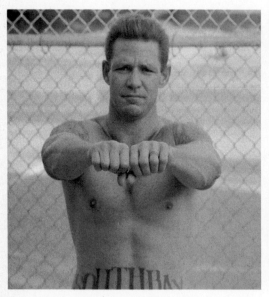
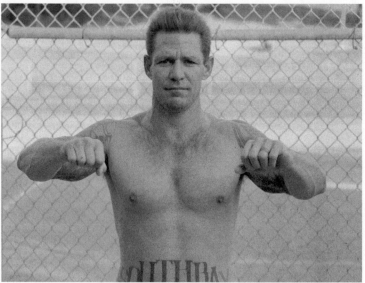

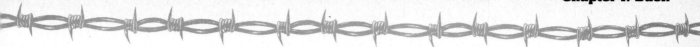

⊘ CEASE AND DESIST

T-bar rows and wide-grip rows, exercises where you pull heavy weights up toward your chest while bent over, put undue stress on your back. However, Chain Breakers will build strength and endurance without the stress since you're standing straight up and not loading your back with heavy weight.

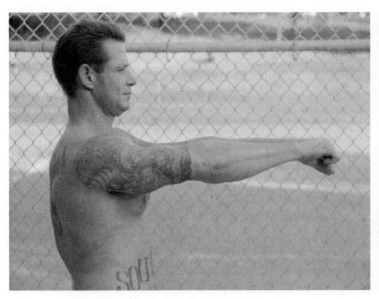 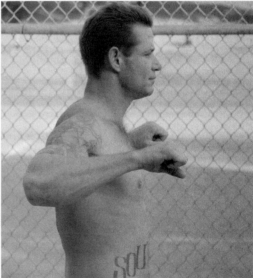

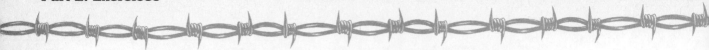

Lawn Mowers (Dumbbell Row)

The "Lawn Mower" is aptly named because you get an accurate visual of how the exercise should look when performed correctly. A Lawn Mower incorporates your lats, biceps, the rear deltoid (the back of your shoulder), and forearm, and because it mimics the movement of picking an item up from the ground it has real-life applications. If you hold your core tight and support your body weight with your abs and lower back, this exercise will allow you to reap many rewards.

To properly do the Lawn Mower, follow the steps below:

1. Hold your prison dumbbell in the hand that will perform the lawn mower movement (the weight of the dumbbell is what makes the exercise effective).

2. Keep your hips and shoulders square to the ground as you pull the weight up from a bent-over position.

3. Stand with your legs either staggered (as shown in the photos) or together.

4. Make sure your elbow stays tucked in close to your torso with your hand just under your chest at the top of the movement.

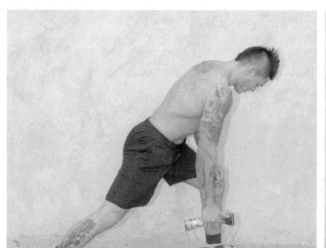

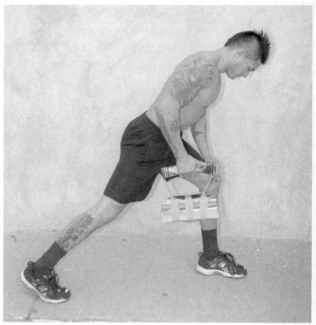

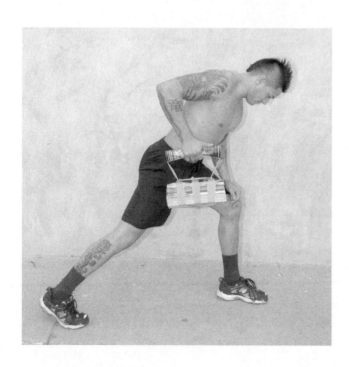

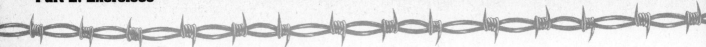

Bent-Over Row

A bent-over row, another great exercise for the mid-traps and rhomboids (located in the middle of your back between your shoulder blades), is similar to a Lawn Mower. During both exercises your chest should be down but slightly higher than your hips and your back needs to be flat. But when doing a bent-over row your hands are now rotated so that the palm of your hand faces back toward your feet and your elbows now stay out from the body. In the images below, notice how the model keeps his back nice and flat while holding / rowing the prison dumbbell:

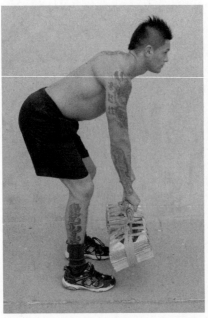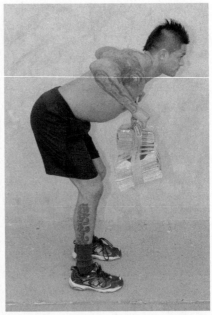

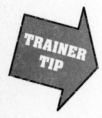

TRAINER TIP

Don't be afraid to pull your tailbone up into the air for this exercise. Your back should not be rounded. Shyness will kill your form during this exercise, so don't be afraid to stick your butt out.

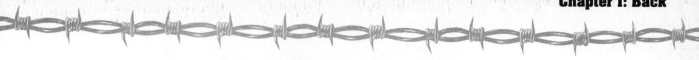

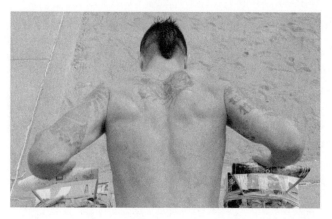

In this photo, please take note of how well the middle of the back is being squeezed for full benefit. When you do this exercise, the contraction of your back should feel like you're trying to hold a piece of paper between your shoulder blades. Don't worry if you feel tension in your lower back as well since it is working to hold your body in the position shown in the corresponding photos.

When you look at the exercise done from the front, you can see how your head should stay down, your chest should be positioned a little higher than your hips, and your elbows should be raised high at the top of the movement before they're lowered back down to your starting position.

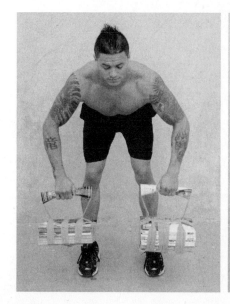
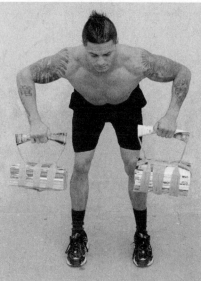
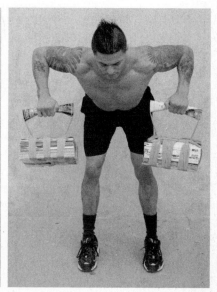

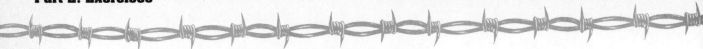

Lower-Back Extensions

This exercise targets your lower back muscle (the *erector spinae*) and other muscles in the back, which are responsible for extending the spine from the lumbar vertebrae (lower spine/back) all the way up to your cervical vertebrae (neck). These muscles work nearly all day long and building them further will keep you sitting/standing up straight correctly without compensational help coming from other muscle groups.

Begin this exercise by lying on the floor facedown, then place your hands on the back of your head with your elbows up, and gently pull your chest off the ground. Slowly lower yourself back down, remembering to breathe.

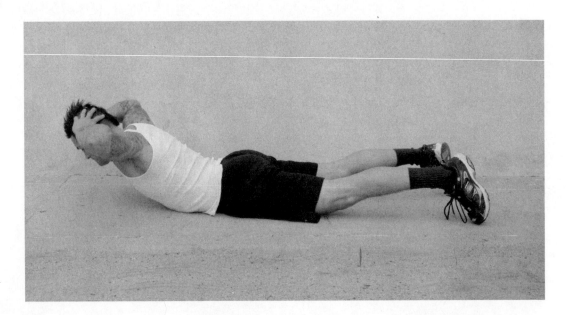

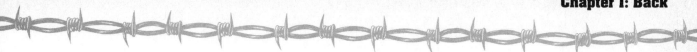

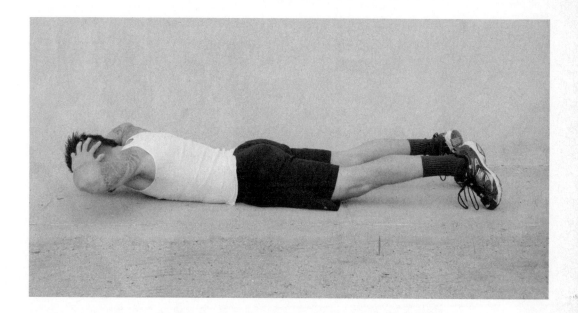

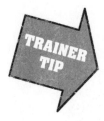

Extend your arms over your head to make the lower back extension even more challenging.

As you pull your chest up really squeeze your glutes (the muscles that make up your rear end). The contraction of your butt will press your hips into the floor and allow for greater extension of the spine.

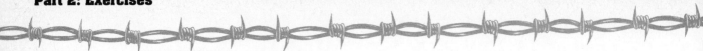

Good Mornings

A Good Morning is a standing lower-back extension that both strengthens your lower back and increases your hamstring flexibility. Perform the exercise slowly as though you were taking a bow on stage with your hands behind your head—lead with your chest while keeping your back flat and legs slightly bent at the knee. Slowly come all the way up while maintaining a straight back and repeat.

Notice how the knees are slightly bent and the back stays flat throughout the entire movement.

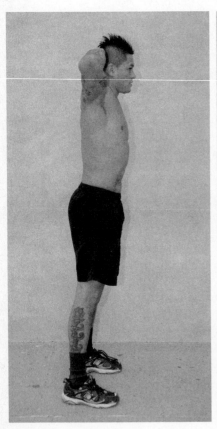
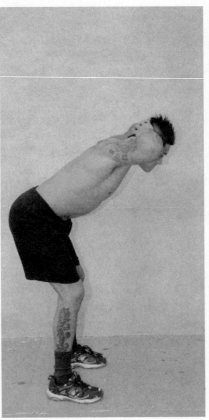
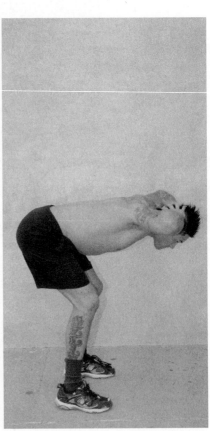

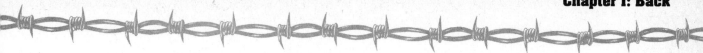

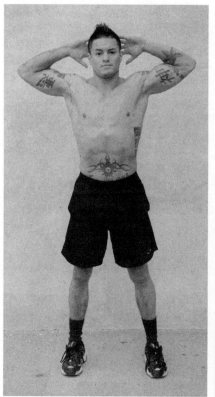
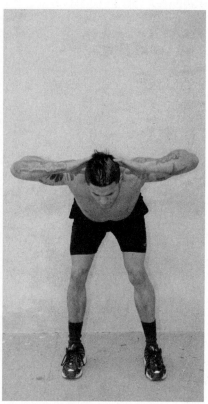

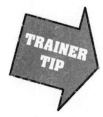

TRAINER TIP

Leg flexibility, especially flexibility in the back of the leg, will help increase range of motion to pick items up off the ground and allow you to step up onto surfaces higher than your knee.

CHAPTER 2

Shoulders

Have you heard the phrase, "carry the weight of the world on your shoulders"? You may not have that much to carry around, but no one can argue against the fact that strong shoulders make life easier. Have you ever tried to store a box high in a closet but weren't quite able to push it in place? Stronger shoulders would have helped. Have you ever been unable to put a suitcase into the overhead compartment of an airplane because it was too heavy? Same solution. The exercises in this section will help to make sure that you can perform the tasks above and more.

The inmates need strong shoulders for different reasons. When attacked, the first instinct for most people is to push the assailant away. A fit inmate can avoid the attack and keep the person at arm's length. But a flabby and weak inmate is in trouble.

If ever you feel an exercise and/or weight is too difficult for you to complete, simply reduce the weight or refrain from doing that particular exercise. Shoulder injuries are painful and take a long time to heal. It's always better to be safe than sorry.

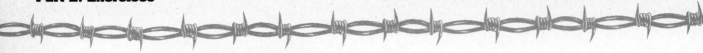

Arm Rotations

Moving your arms in circles both forward and backward is a great endurance exercise and will warm up your shoulders to help prevent injury. You may think that this exercise seems too easy, but once you try to perform 200 rotations without stopping you'll see just how effective it actually is. Even when raising your arms high over your head, be sure to keep your shoulder blades pressed down to maintain joint stability, which will help avoid rotator cuff issues.

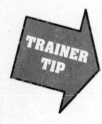

TRAINER TIP

Perform arm rotations while walking to make your workout more intense or to make a warm-up more thorough.

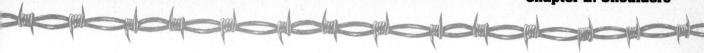

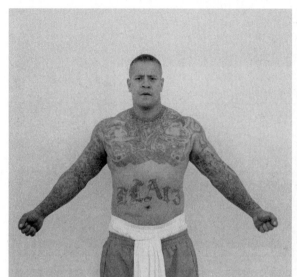

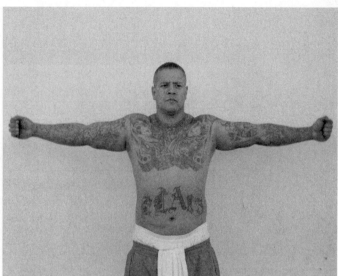

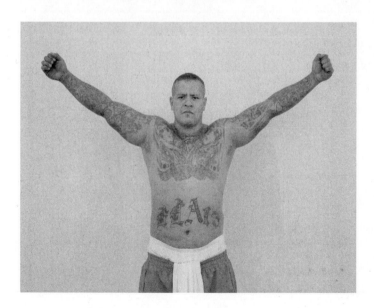

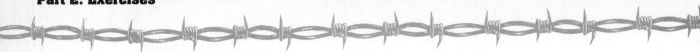

Butterfly

You can work both the middle part of your back between your shoulder blades and your entire shoulder by performing the Butterfly. Start with your arms straight out in front of you at shoulder height. Pull them back as far as you can while keeping them straight and at shoulder level. Then raise your arms together over your head (keeping them straight). Bring your arms back down in front at shoulder height and repeat.

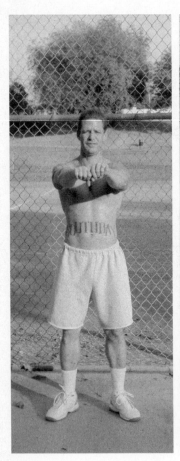
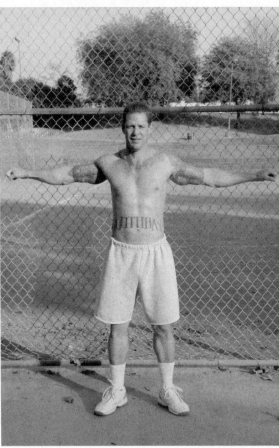
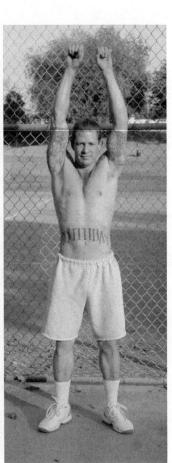

Be sure to squeeze between your shoulder blades as you pull your arms back. This movement and muscle contraction will work the back of the shoulders and the middle of your trapezius (the muscle in the middle of your upper back, between your shoulder blades) while stretching out your chest. Holding your arms up also works the deltoid (the one and only muscle that makes up your shoulder).

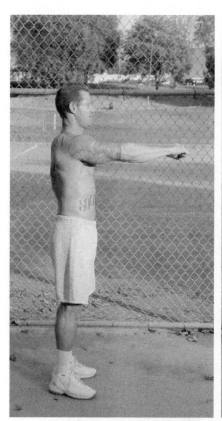
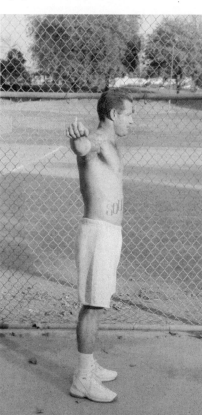
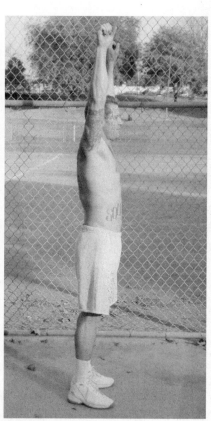

⊘ CEASE AND DESIST

The Butterfly is a great alternative to the reverse dumbbell fly/rear delt fly, a bent-over exercise during which dumbbells are raised with a straight arm away from the body, forming a large "T" with the arms and torso. These exercises can put a lot of stress on your back since they're performed in a bent-over position. The Butterfly strengthens the back of the shoulder just as well as these gym-based movements without putting the back at risk.

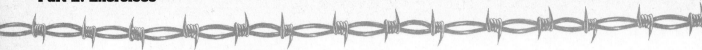

Upright Row

With your hands together using an overhand grip, take your prison dumbbell and raise the weight up, bending your elbows and lifting your arms to a point where your hands are directly under your chin. You'll feel the burn from this exercise in the top part of your shoulders.

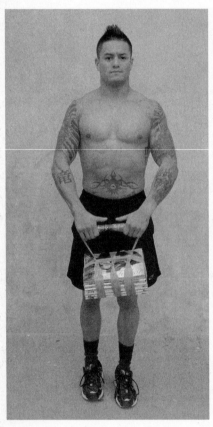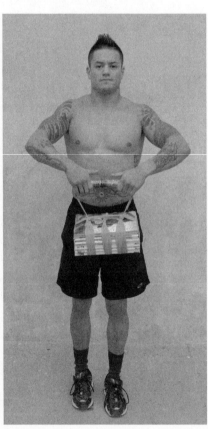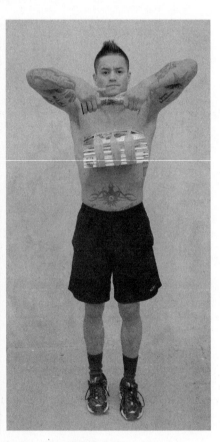

Once you have your arms raised, slowly lower them back to their starting position before doing another repetition. While performing an Upright Row it's important to keep your shoulders back. If your shoulders are slouched forward you increase your risk of injury during the exercise.

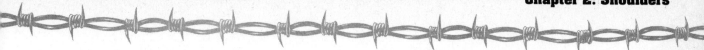

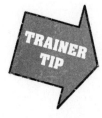

Instead of adding more magazines to your prison dumbbell when exercises become too easy, start performing the movement with one hand so you don't have to take apart your dumbbell or buy heavier weights.

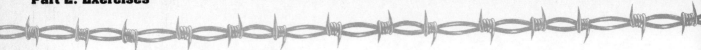

Curl and Press

This is a great combination exercise that gives the arms a complete workout. You're simply doing curls for the biceps and adding an overhead press. The pressing movement works the shoulder and, since the weight you're using needs to be light for you to perform curls during the first part of the movement, you won't hurt your back. For this exercise, you'll need to use your prison dumbbell to add the needed resistance for strength training. Start by holding the magazines (not the dumbbell handle) or the strips that hold the magazines together. Curl the weight up toward your chest, moving only the forearm up, hinging at the elbow. Then press the weight overhead while keeping your back straight and abdominals held tight.

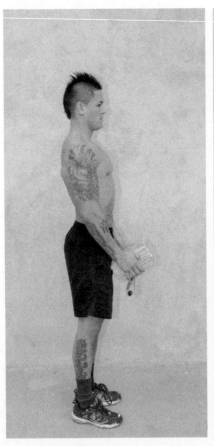 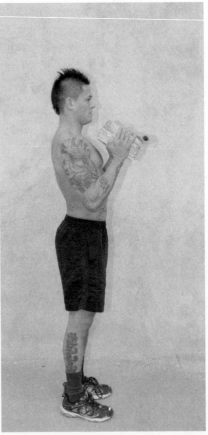

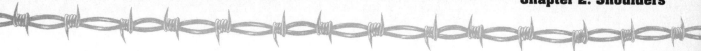

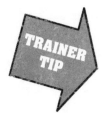

TRAINER TIP

Whenever you perform an exercise that requires you to move weight over your head, always be sure to keep your body supported with a tight stomach. If you feel any discomfort in your lower back, either use a lighter weight and see if that helps or immediately stop doing the exercise.

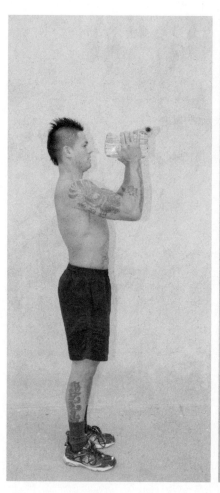
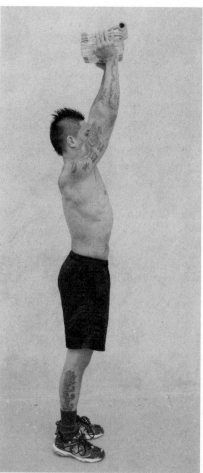

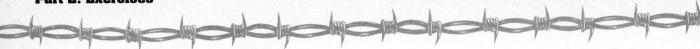

Lateral Raises

To work the middle of your shoulders, start by grabbing your prison dumbbell(s). Stand with them at your side and raise your arm(s) to shoulder height while keeping your arm straight. Once the dumbbell is shoulder high, slowly lower the weight back to the starting position.

A little bit of weight goes a long way with this exercise, so start small, be patient, and work your way up.

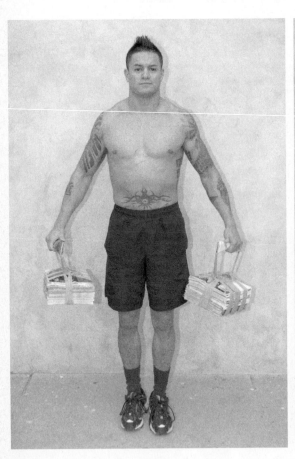
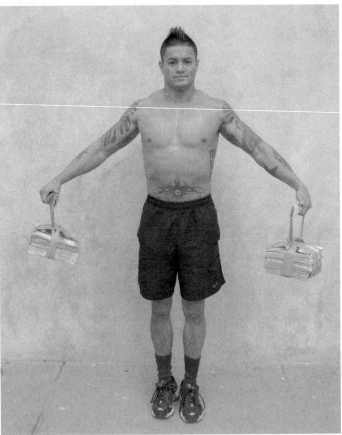

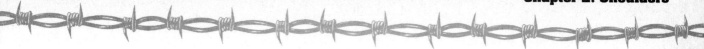

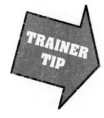

Don't lean away from the weight to compensate for it being too heavy. If you find yourself leaning back, reduce the weight.

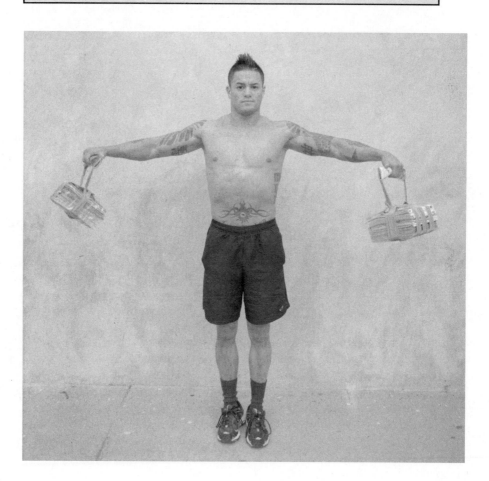

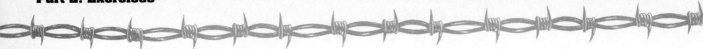

Front Raise

Grab your dumbbell with an overhand grip and stand with your feet shoulder-width apart. Raise the weight up straight in front of you to shoulder level before lowering it at a very controlled rate.

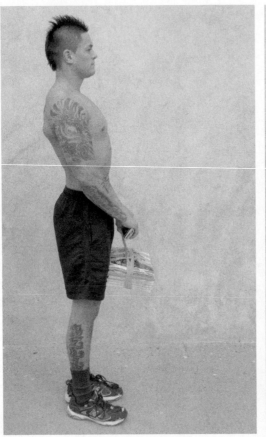 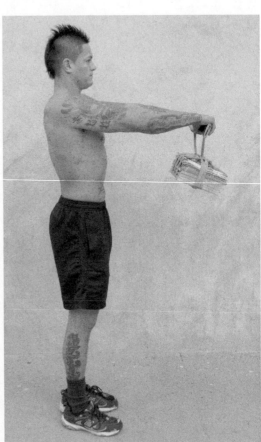

Front raises can be done with one hand or two and are great for developing the front part of the shoulder.

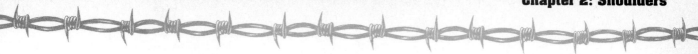

Shrugs

This movement is often put with shoulder exercises even though it works the uppermost part of your back (the part that slopes down from your neck to the top of your shoulder) more than anything. In order to do a shrug correctly all you have to do is hold your dumbbells at your sides and elevate your shoulders up toward your ears. Slowly lower your shoulders to a normal resting position before beginning your next repetition.

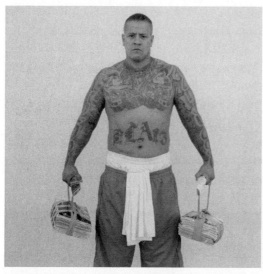
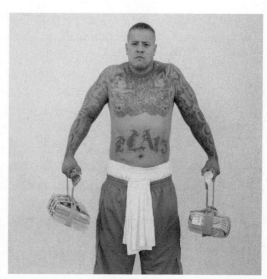
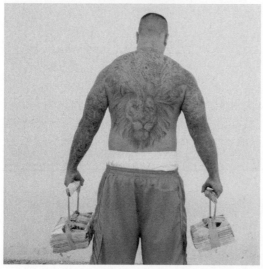
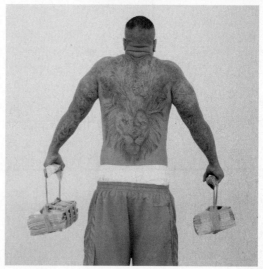

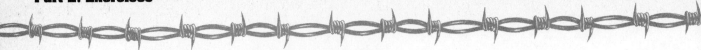

Handstand Push-Up

The most difficult shoulder exercise you'll ever try is the handstand push-up. In addition to using your shoulders to push up your body weight you are also stabilizing your body with at least eight different muscles in the shoulder complex.

Start the handstand push-up by placing your hands on the ground about six inches away from a wall. With your arms straight, kick your legs up so they can balance against the wall. From this inverted position, slowly lower your body down until your head is three inches from the ground before pressing back up. The pressing motion needs to be explosive and requires a lot of strength. If you can't perform this movement at least three times, wait until you've developed the necessary strength to do so before you try a full set.

It's wise to use a sturdy wall for balance while performing this exercise. Make sure there is nothing around the area where you're doing handstand push-ups so you don't hurt yourself or others who might be standing around you. The last thing you want to do is come down on something hard or sharp after finishing a set.

🚫 CEASE AND DESIST

Overhead barbell presses, overhead dumbbell presses, and Arnold presses—where you push weights over your head while either sitting or standing—can all lead to injury if performed with too much weight or with improper form. If the weight is too heavy you may find yourself leaning back, trying desperately not to drop the weight, or you may fail to complete the exercise. Your lower back will thank you more and more as you eliminate the overhead exercises listed.

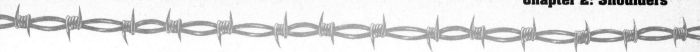

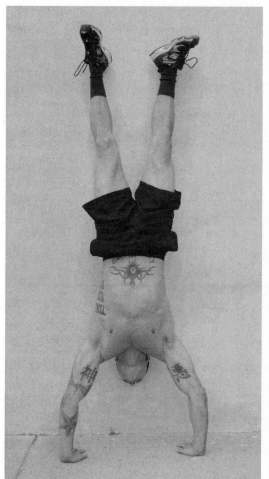 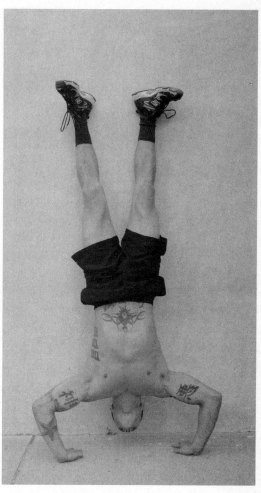

You may have to practice before perfecting this exercise, so don't give up if you can't get it right the first time.

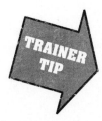

TRAINER
TIP

You've heard the phrase "Quality over quantity"? An exercise is only as effective as the quality of the movement. Ten push-ups with great form are much better than thirty push-ups with lousy form. This principle applies to all exercises.

CHAPTER 3

Chest

You may have an image in your head of a stereotypically muscular inmate: He has a huge chest—so big, in fact, that his extraordinarily tight chest muscles cause the bone in his upper arm to rotate forward, which makes him slouch like a lower-order primate. This internal rotation of the upper arm is common among many gym-going males and happens because the muscles in the back aren't strong enough to balance out the body. The simple way to correct this muscular imbalance is to strengthen the middle of your upper back (trapezius), as we discussed in the last chapter, and stretch the chest. So let's take a look at some of these chest exercises—most of which involve some variation of the push-up—but be careful to find balance in your workout routine, especially when it comes to this part of the body.

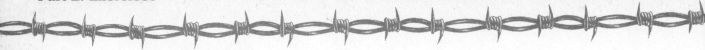

Push-Ups

The most time-tested exercise for chest workouts is the push-up. When you complete push-ups you work a lot more than the chest muscles; you also activate the transverse abdominus (the innermost abdominal muscle), serratus anterior (the muscle that looks like fake ribs just below the outer part of your chest), the triceps (the back of the arm), and the deltoid (shoulder).

To perform a push-up:

1. Lay on the ground face down with your hands shoulder-width apart. Keep your chest over your hands, your legs and back straight, and your feet on the ground. Only your hands and feet should be on the ground.

2. Inhale as you lower your body down evenly and in a controlled fashion. Your hips and chest should go down together and your back needs to remain straight (you should come within two inches from the ground without touching).

3. Exhale as you press your body up from the ground. Your hips, torso, and legs should move up together until your arms are straight at the top.

4. Repeat steps 1–3 until you've done your required number of reps.

Changing your hand positions or the positions of your hips and other body parts changes the focus of the exercise. On the following pages, you'll find multiple variations and descriptions of how to use these exercises to get the most from your workout.

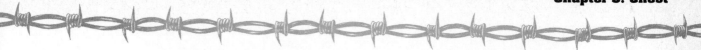

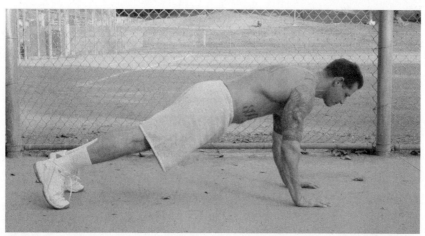

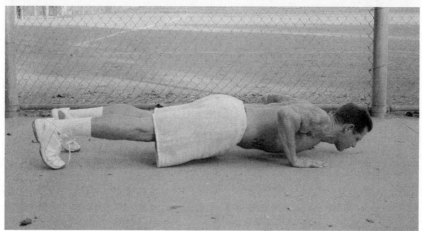

⊘ CEASE AND DESIST

The flat bench press (Barbell or Dumbbell), incline press (Bb or Db), and decline press (Bb or Db), where you lie on your back and push hundreds of pounds away from your chest, all have limited functional value. These exercises also have injured thousands of shoulders, as men and women often use bad form. Chest muscles tightened by these exercises also affect posture by rotating your shoulders forward, creating that unattractive slouch.

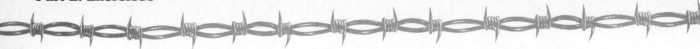

Diamond Push-Ups

This particular kind of push-up places the emphasis of the exercise on the triceps (the back of the upper arm), the center of the chest closest to the sternum, and the front of the shoulder (anterior deltoid). Place your hands close together with the tips of your index fingers and thumbs touching. Keep your chest over your hands and your elbows close to your side and complete a push-up. You should feel the difference between a traditional push-up and a diamond push-up immediately.

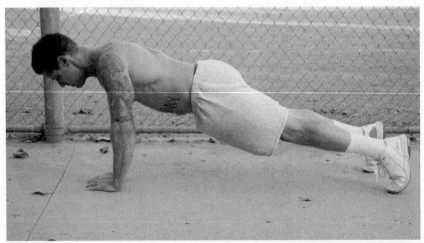

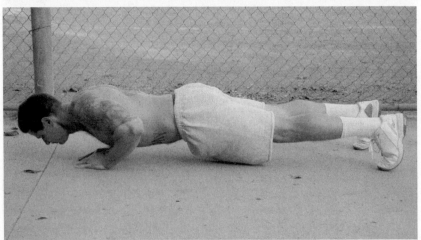

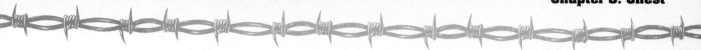

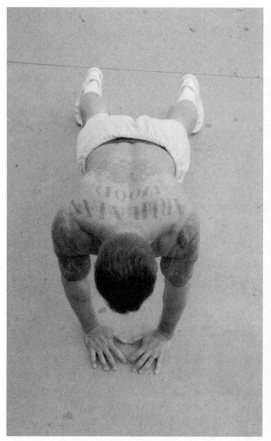 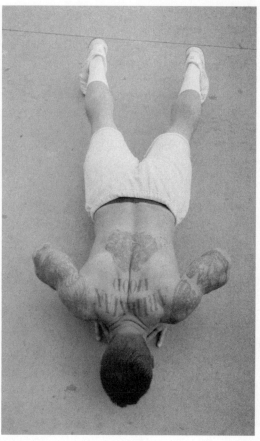

You can see in the photo just how close your hands are during this particular type of push-up.

🚫 CEASE AND DESIST

Avoid the close-grip bench press, where you lie on your back and push dangerous amounts of weight over your body with your hands closer than shoulder-width apart. This shoulder-busting exercise is just waiting to take your rotator cuff hostage.

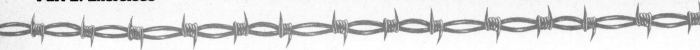

"Celly"/Partner Push-Up

Before you get started you need to find a workout partner for this particular push-up. The extra body weight of your workout partner both adds more resistance to your chest and makes your core work much harder to keep your body straight and moving as a unit.

To perform a celly push-up, get into the normal push-up position. Then have your workout partner align your two bodies; his shoulder blades will touch your shoulder blades, his buttocks will align with yours, his back will touch your back, and his legs will rest on your legs. Have your partner cross his arms over his chest in order to avoid swinging and touching the ground. Keep in mind that you need to hold your partner's weight safely off the ground before you even begin a push-up. Once you're ready slowly lower your body down within three inches of the ground before exploding up as you exhale.

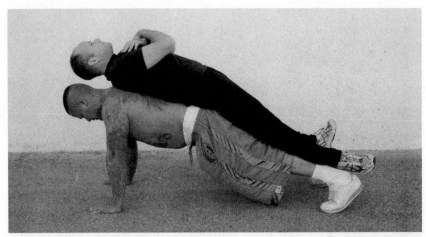

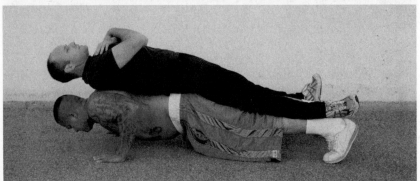

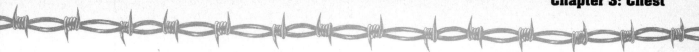

Incline Push-Up

Working the upper part of your chest during a push-up is as simple as elevating your feet on a chair, a bed, bleachers, a bench, etc. Be sure to keep your head up in order to increase your range of motion.

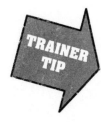

TRAINER TIP

Push-ups are great exercises because they are "closed-chain" movements. Simply put, closed-chain means the end of your arm is in a fixed position, which helps prevent injury because it is a much more stable exercise.

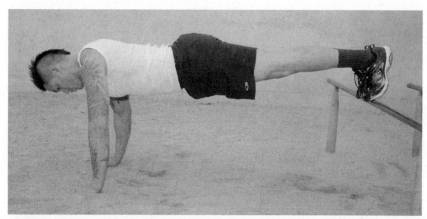

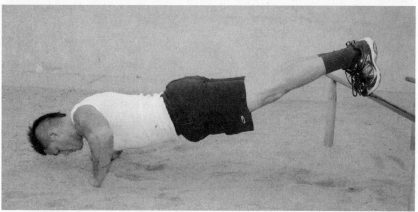

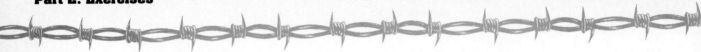

Wide Push-Up

If you want to blast the lateral part of your chest (the part closest to your armpit) and the lower part of the chest (pec minor), position your hands twice as wide as you normally would and keep your fingers pointed outward. Complete the push-up and you will feel a significant difference between this exercise and a traditional push-up; rather than feeling the burn in the middle of the chest, you'll feel it toward the outside of the chest, closer to the armpit and shoulder.

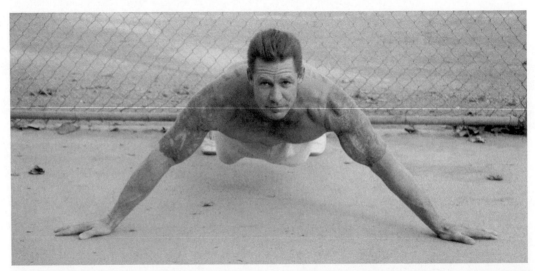

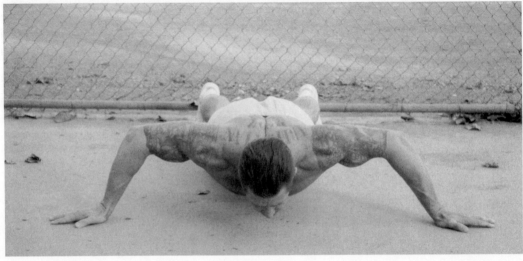

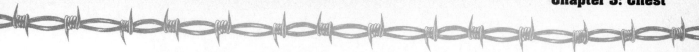

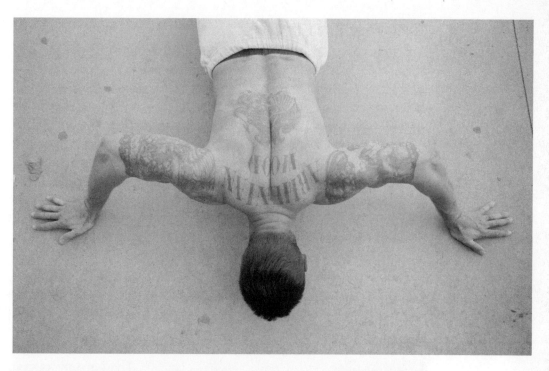

⊘ CEASE AND DESIST

Cable flies and cable crossovers are two more exercises that can pull your shoulder into harm's way quicker than you can say "It wasn't me, officer." These exercises, which use unstable pulleys attached to weight stacks, have you pushing handles toward the middle of your body while keeping your arms straight. Too often people perform these exercises with bad form. Avoid them by doing wide push-ups.

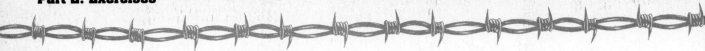

Plyometric Push-Up

Plyometric exercises are explosive in nature; they require your body to burst off the ground into the air and then return to its starting position in rapid succession. You have to generate a lot of force in order to propel your body either off the ground or off the object bearing your weight. But these push-ups are challenging not only because you have to push your body off the ground (or a bar, as in the photos) but also because you have to decelerate your body in order to keep your chest from slamming onto the ground or into the bar from which you just pushed off.

To do the Plyometric Push-Up:

1. Keep your eyes on your destination. You will explode off the ground/ bar as you exhale and be temporarily airborne.

2. "Catch" your own body. Your hands will land back on the ground/ bar. You must keep your elbows bent in order to avoid injuring your wrists and elbows.

3. Hold the rest of your body as stiff as you can since gravity will be pulling you down. You must use your upper body and core strength to prevent your body from falling to the ground.

4. Once you're safely back to the starting position you have to explode back off the ground to keep your momentum shifting up and down, making the exercise challenging and effective.

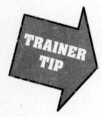

TRAINER TIP

If you're new to exercise you should wait a while before trying plyometric movements. Be sure to perfect regular forms of push-ups and lunges; then, once you can do the traditional exercises in your sleep, you can move on to "plyos."

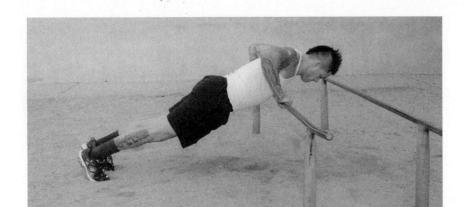

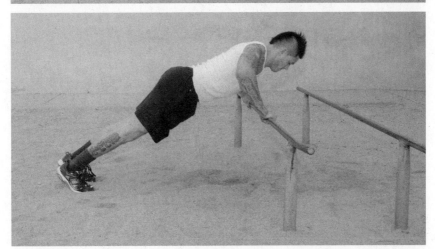

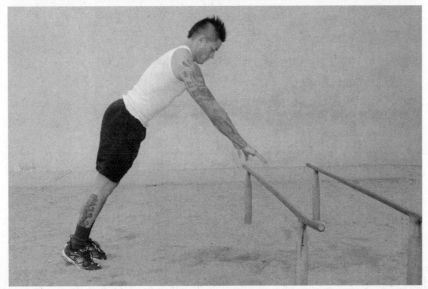

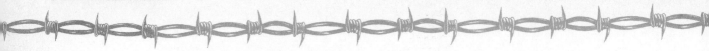

Push-Up with Hip Extension

Another small enhancement that makes a push-up more of a challenge is the hip extension. When pushing your body up lift up one leg with the knee straight. This movement challenges your core by forcing you to balance as well as work the glutes (your rear end/butt muscles) and hamstrings. Be sure to alternate legs so you complete an equal number of hip extensions during your set of push-ups.

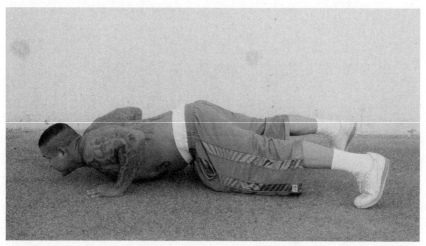

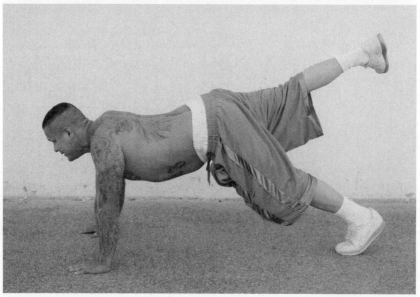

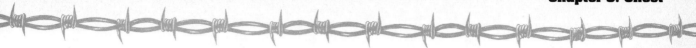

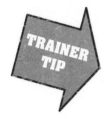

If you do an even number of sets for the hip-extension push-ups, try a full set on one leg before switching legs for your next set. This adds another layer of difficulty to this exercise and is a good change to make for continued results.

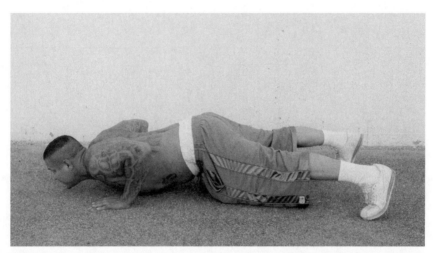

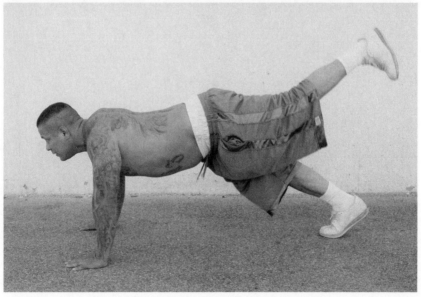

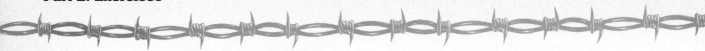

Staggered Hand Push-Ups

Make your push-ups interesting by staggering your hand position during sets of push-ups. Place one hand further in front of you as though you are crawling and keep the second hand in its traditional position. The hand placed closer to your torso will do more work, helping to build the chest since it is experiencing more resistance. As always, be sure to do an equal number of push-ups on each side.

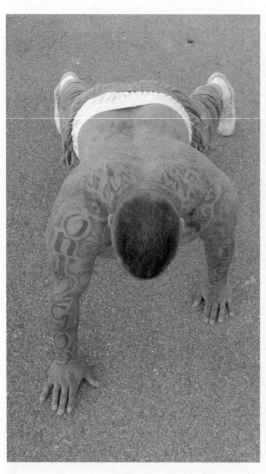 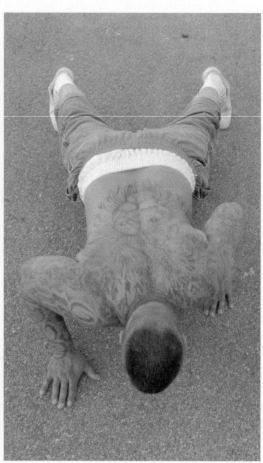

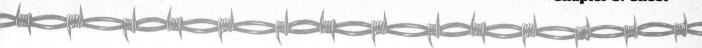

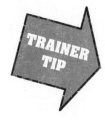

When performing a staggered push-up correctly you will resemble Spider-Man crawling along a wall or a prisoner scaling a wall in an attempt to escape.

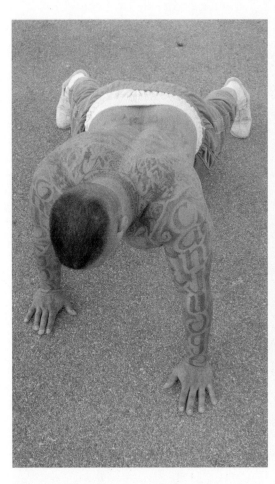

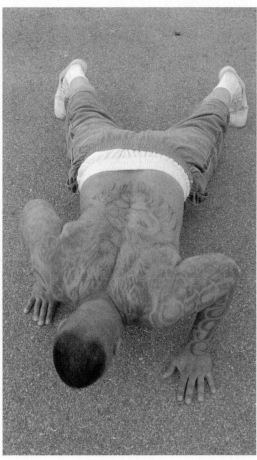

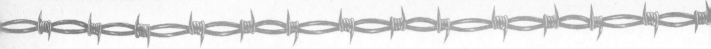

Dumbbell Fly

While most of the chest exercises we've discussed have been push-up–related, there are other exercises you can do to work your chest. The dumbbell fly is one of them. While on your back (using a bench or chair or lying on the ground) and with your dumbbells in either one or both hands over your chest, bend your elbows slightly while opening your arms. Exhale as you reverse the movement by lifting the weight and closing your arms. This "fly" movement will work the middle part of your chest, closest to the sternum.

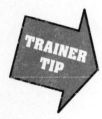

TRAINER TIP

Think of this exercise as hugging a tree. Your arms need to open wide with a slight bend, so the visual of being a literal tree hugger should help you get the movement down with good form.

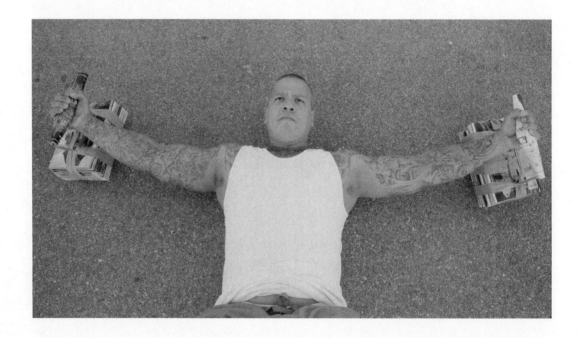

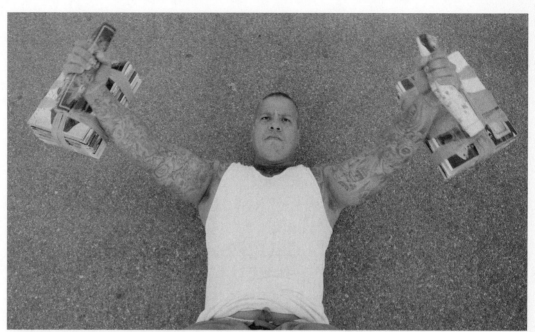

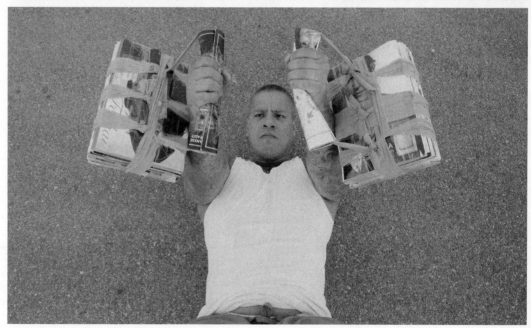

CHAPTER 4

Legs

Leg strengthening is too often ignored by men (remember the chest-heavy inmate described in the previous chapter?), which is a mistake because, for most people, the hips and legs account for over half of all body weight. So if you fail to train your legs, you are missing an opportunity to really help rid your body of unwanted fat and get truly ripped since the increased testosterone produced by additional leg mass will help you develop muscles everywhere else. The increase in muscle mass will also boost your metabolic rate, making it easier to lose both fat and inches around your waist. In turn you'll burn more calories when your body is at rest throughout the day. Note: This change occurs in both men and women, but women shouldn't worry about "bulking up" since their bodies can't produce enough testosterone to get bigger.

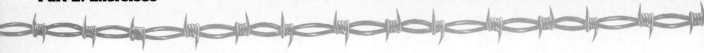

Squats

The bread-and-butter exercise of any leg routine is the basic squat. Here are some tips:

1. Keep your knees from moving laterally (side to side) as you sit down into the squat.

2. Keep your chest high and shoulders back as you lower your body down.

3. Don't be afraid to sit back during a squat.

4. Push through your feet evenly with your toes and heels.

5. You'll notice that the model in the photo has his hands up under his chin. However, you should feel free to keep your hands where you feel most comfortable as long as your shoulders are down and back.

⊘ CEASE AND DESIST

Stay away from barbell squats and front squats. Once again, these exercises (squats performed with a loaded barbell held across the back of the neck and top of the chest, respectively) place a lot of stress on your back, neck, and arms. Keep them out of your routine and your back will thank you later when you're old and up for parole.

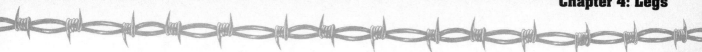

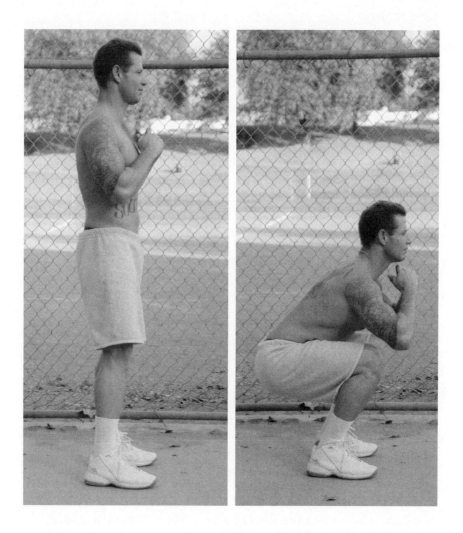

In this photo you can see the good form, which includes an impressive range of motion.

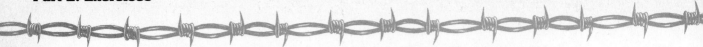

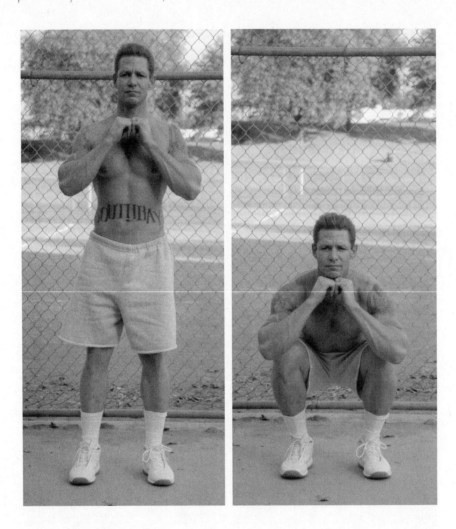

Notice how the feet and knees continue to point forward even in this deep squat.

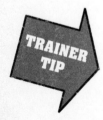

TRAINER TIP

If you have trouble maintaining good form during a squat, try sitting down on a chair and then stand up again. As you improve, sit on lower objects until you can perform a squat without a "safety net."

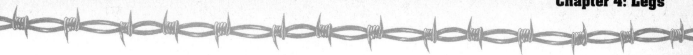

Bulgarian/Romanian Squats

Eastern Europeans must be tough sons-of-bitches because this exercise is tough. A Bulgarian/Romanian squat puts all of the focus of the squat on your front leg. With your back foot resting on an elevated surface (a bench, chair, bar, etc.) make sure that nearly all of your weight is shifted forward to get the most out of this surprisingly difficult exercise.

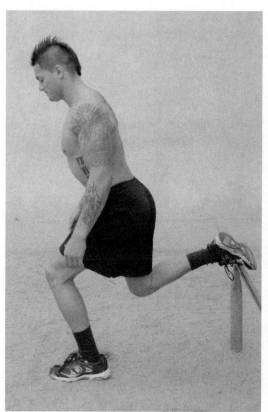 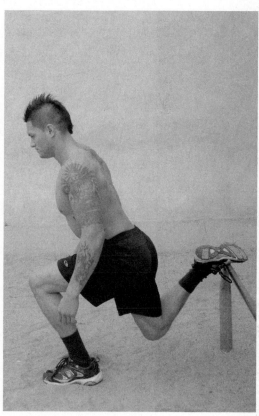

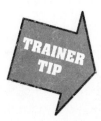

Vitamin C helps reduce soreness. Try grapefruit or an orange.

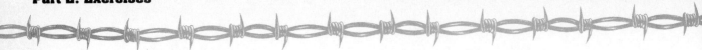

Pistol Squat

Pistol squats are even more difficult than Bulgarian/Romanian squats. They're so challenging because they require a lot more effort and support from the core, since you are not resting your elevated leg on anything around you. This exercise demands tremendous lower-body strength in addition to good balance and flexibility.

While doing pistol squats, let your arms extend forward in order to maintain balance. You'll feel your back engage as the muscles that line your spine work to keep you upright. You also need to draw your abdominals in and keep them tight in order to stay balanced and avoid injury.

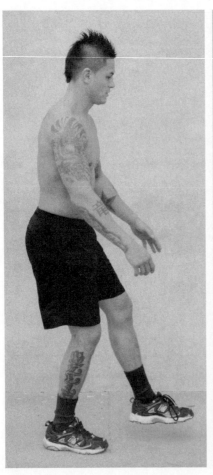
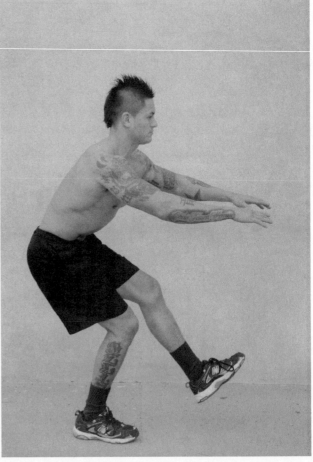

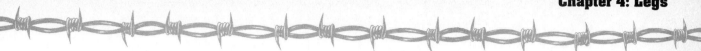

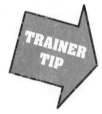

TRAINER TIP

Sitting on a bench or chair is an excellent way to start, but if you have the necessary strength and flexibility, try a pistol squat without anything underneath to catch you as you lower yourself toward the ground.

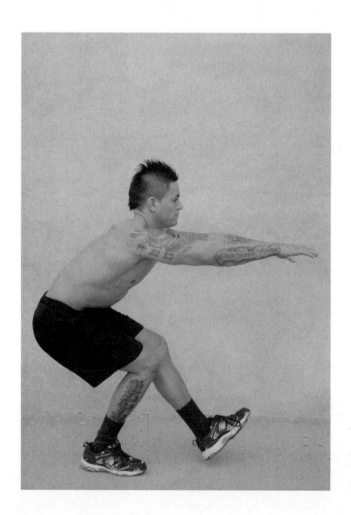

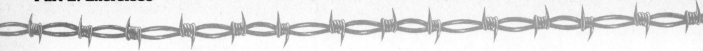

Jump Squats

There isn't a lot of mystery in the content of this exercise given its name. A jump squat is exactly what it sounds like: A vertical jump where you land into a squat. Here are a few tips to keep in mind while doing this exercise:

1. Land softly by squatting as soon as you feel your toes touch the ground.

2. You can have the option of swinging your arms up as you explode off your feet into the jump. This arm motion will get your momentum moving up, taking a bit of strain away from your legs.

3. Keep your head up when you land; this will help you keep your balance.

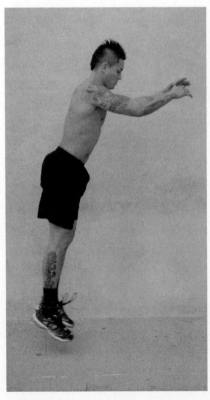
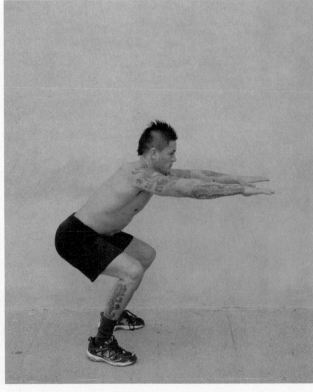

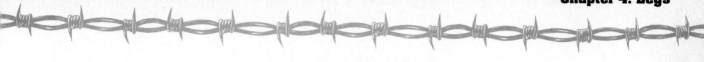

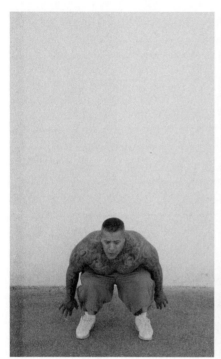

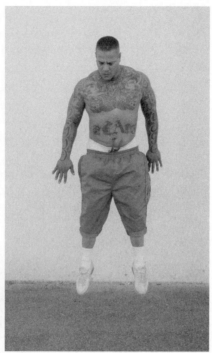

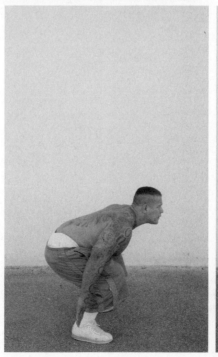

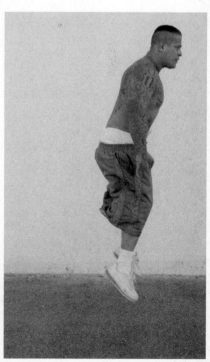

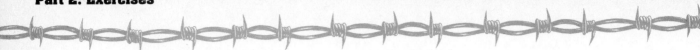

Lunges

Think of a lunge as a single-leg squat with a kick-stand; you're now just using your front leg to push more of your own weight and your back leg to help you balance yourself throughout the movement. Lunges can be done in place (static lunges), forward and back (alternating lunges), from one point to another (walking lunges), or from side to side (lateral lunges). All of these lunge variations work the front of the thigh, the hamstrings, and the rear end, with emphasis shifting depending on the exercise and alignment of the body. Static lunges emphasize the butt, lateral lunges work your inner and outer thighs a bit more, and walking lunges are more difficult because you're moving your body more.

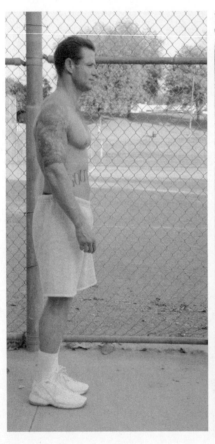
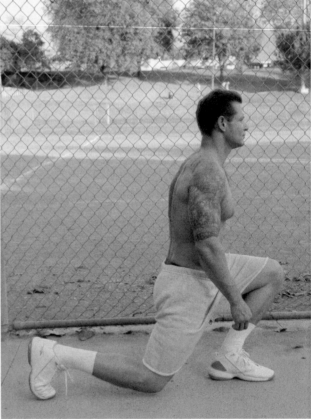

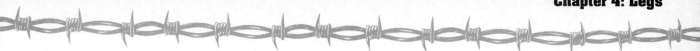

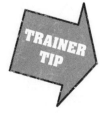

Start with static lunges (they're easiest). Move on to alternating lunges second. Walking lunges are probably the hardest, especially if you decide to add the weight of prison dumbbells.

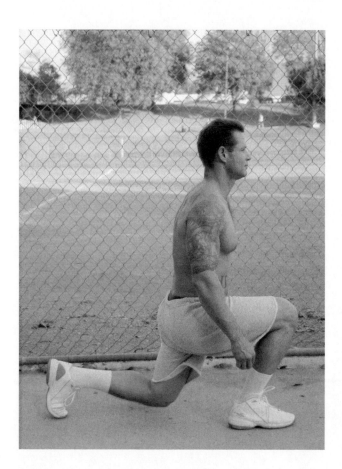

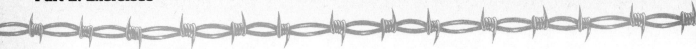

Plyometric Lunges

In the same way that plyometric push-ups help you power-up your arms, the plyometric lunge helps you develop explosive power in your legs. With this lunge, your body actually leaves the ground. It is essentially a jump from a deep knee bend and staggered leg position. When jumping off the ground, be sure to keep your legs working as a synchronized unit: Both feet should push off with the same amount of force and land at the same time to ensure that landings and take-offs are smooth and effective.

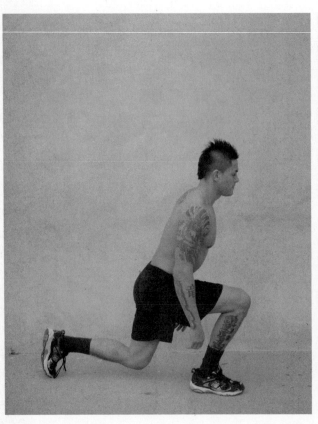
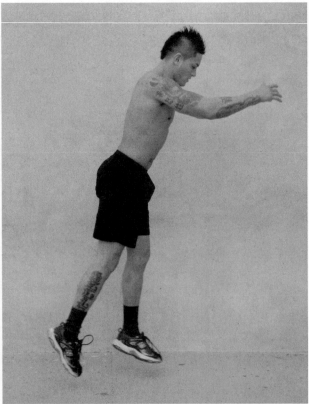

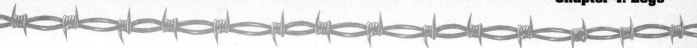

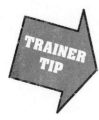

Switching your legs in the air is a great way to make the plyometric lunge even more difficult. In order to complete a switch, you must move your legs in a "scissor" motion the moment you leave the ground. At the peak of the jump your legs should be together and they should begin to separate as you descend with the force of gravity. Keep a slight bend in the knee to avoid injury when landing. Continue switching with each successive repetition until you complete the set.

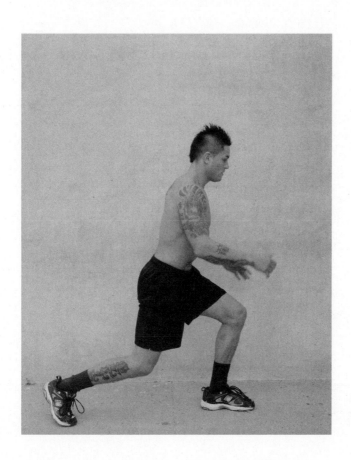

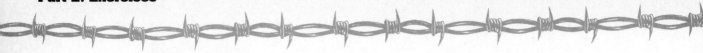

Step-Ups

Step-ups are exactly what they sound like; you step up onto a surface and then step back down. The higher the surface, the harder the step-up. You should start low and work your way higher and higher. A standard step on a flight of stairs is eight inches in height. Find something that suits your current level of fitness (the model is using his prison dumbbell as a step) and get started. If you want to make the exercise more difficult for both your core and sense of balance lift your knee at the top of a step-up.

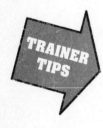

TRAINER TIPS

✱ This exercise is very useful since it strengthens your leg with the functional step movement. Combined with an upper-body exercise, step-ups really do a great job of burning calories and making workouts more time-efficient.

✱ Step-ups and/or lunges are killer exercises. They use a minimum of nine muscles in the leg, which burns a lot of calories. When combined with bicep curls, lateral raises, front raises, and hammer curls you have an exercise that burns calories, builds muscle, and improves your cardiovascular health because it is so damn hard.

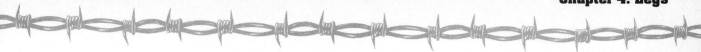

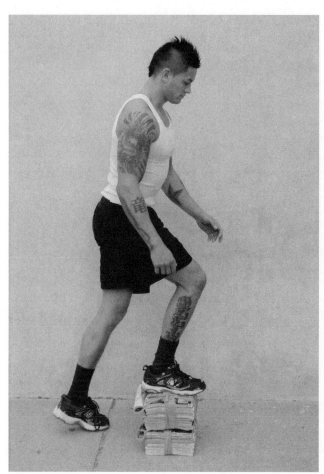

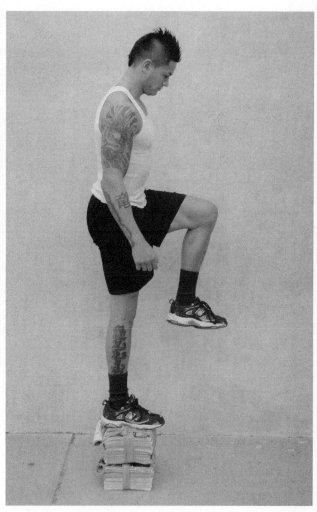

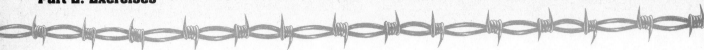

Step-Ups with a Twist

To put a spin on the normal step-up try holding your hands behind your head and twisting at the top of the step-up to give your obliques (the sides of the abdomen) a great workout. Remember to focus on turning your shoulders in order to get the best range of motion. That in turn will engage more muscles for a greater result.

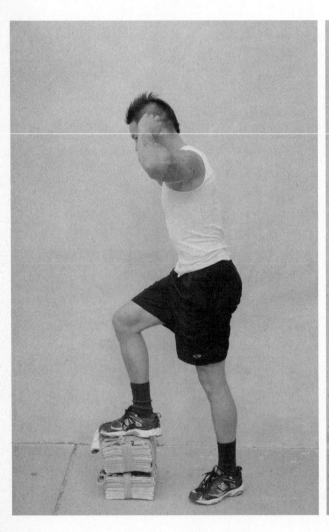 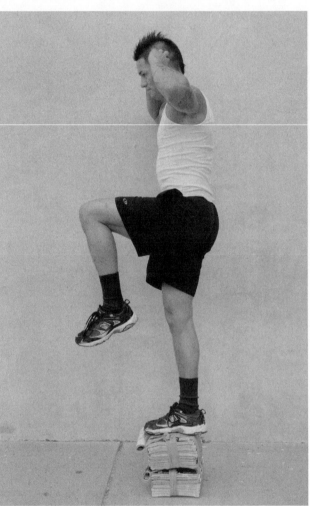

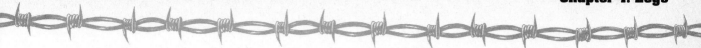

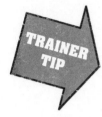

TRAINER TIP

Always eat protein with a carbohydrate after a workout; this combination helps restore energy sources to your muscles quickly.

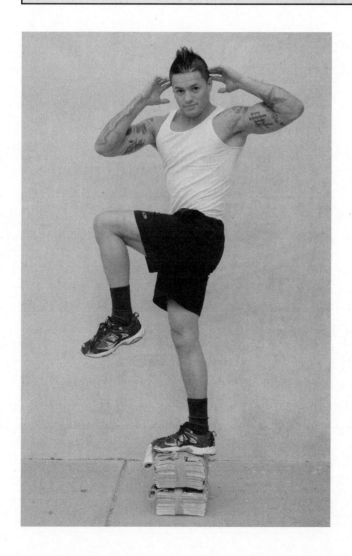

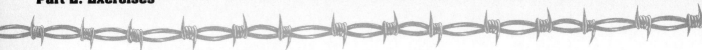

Palm Kicks

Palm kicks (lovingly called "Frankensteins" by some) are a great way to work your legs while increasing your hamstring flexibility. Simply squat while holding your arms in front of you and kick your left hand with your right foot as you stand up. Squat again and kick your right hand with your left foot. That two-squat/two-kick cycle equals one repetition.

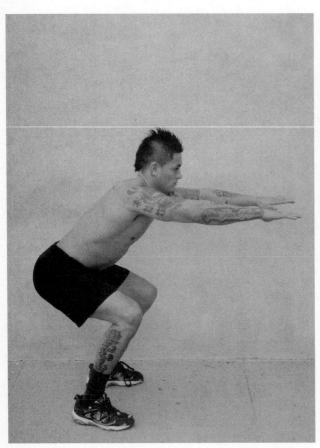 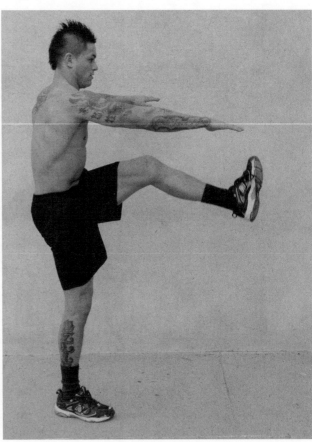

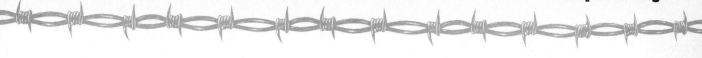

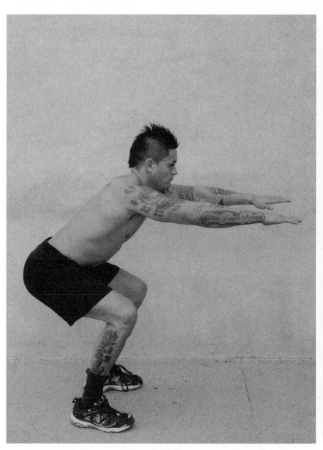

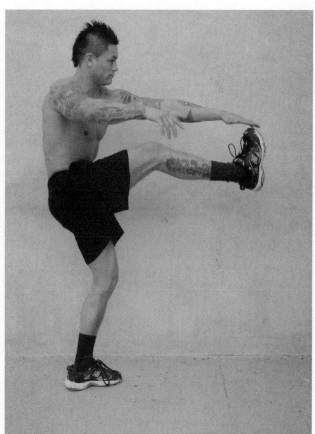

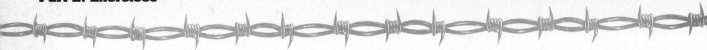

This exercise incorporates several muscle groups, making it a very effective and time-efficient movement.

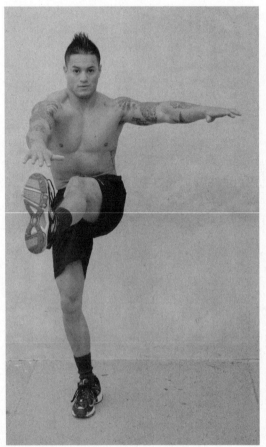 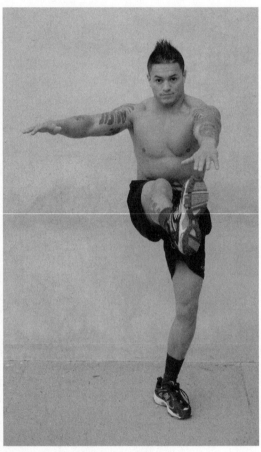

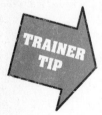

TRAINER TIP

Remember to hydrate. Nothing can affect a workout in a negative way more than a lack of fluids. Be sure to drink plenty of water!

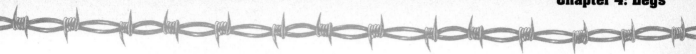

Calf Raises

This exercise is a great way to work your gastrocnemius (calves) because you're pressing your body up onto your toes with just that small muscle. To get into position imagine that you're waiting to get patted down after being pulled over by the cops, with your hands on the top of the car. Be sure to keep your legs straight as you use your calves to lift your body up onto the tips of your toes.

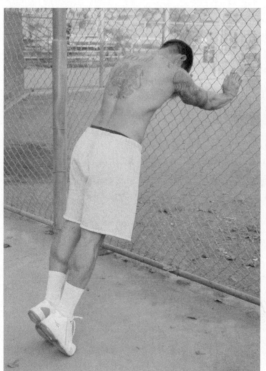 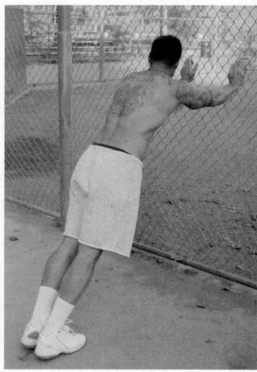

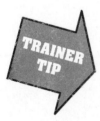

TRAINER TIP

Calf raises can be done on an elevated surface—such as a stairway in your home—to increase your range of motion. When you're lowering your body, allow your heel to pass lower than the edge of the surface where you're standing to make the exercise more effective.

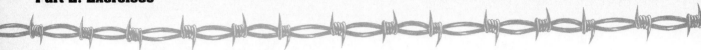

Cherry Pickers

The simple Cherry Picker is a great way to both develop flexibility in your hamstrings (back of the leg) and to increase your hip mobility. With your legs spread wide, use both hands to reach down to your left leg, then reach over to the middle, and then over to the right leg before coming all the way up and slamming your tightened abs with your fists. This exercise is also a great way to measure your increased range of motion as you perform them over a period of time.

If you're not quite able to touch the ground or your feet, work your way up to it. See how long it takes to develop that kind of flexibility. If you're already flexible enough to touch your toes and the ground, try to get your palms flat on the ground during each phase of the exercise.

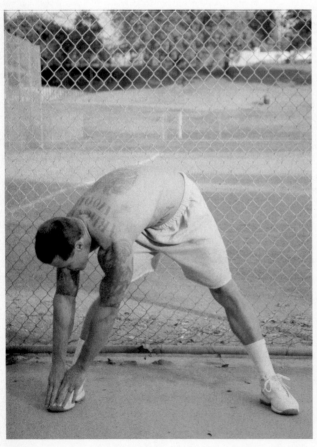
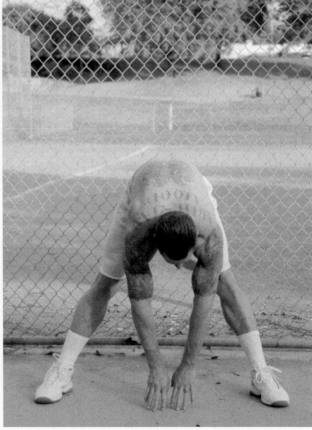

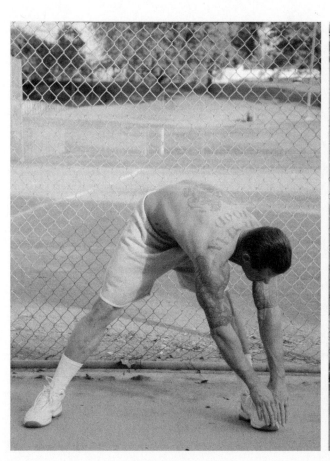 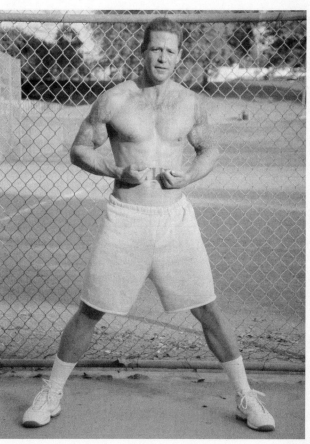

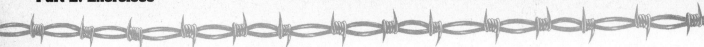

Belly Busters

"Belly Buster" is a terrible misnomer. This exercise is much better at improving hamstring flexibility. From a standing position, reach down to touch your toes before reaching into the air with your arms straight up and your feet firmly on the ground. As you put your arms down, slam your fists into your stomach just as you do when performing Cherry Pickers.

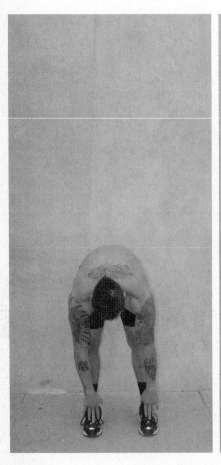
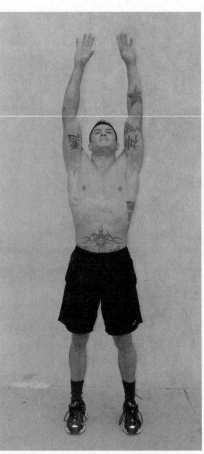
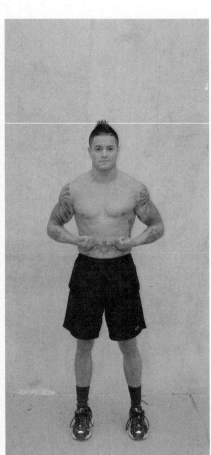

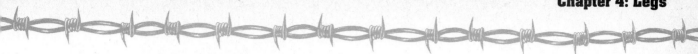

Windmills

A cousin to the Cherry Picker that will also improve your flexibility is the Windmill. It differs from the Cherry Picker in that you're doing more of a rotational movement while keeping your torso flexed downwards throughout most of the exercise. With a stance wider than your shoulders, reach down and touch your left foot or left shin with your right hand while keeping your legs straight. Stay down in this position and turn your shoulders to touch your right foot or right shin with your left hand. This is a great exercise to strengthen back muscles, stretch your hamstrings, and develop core strength as well.

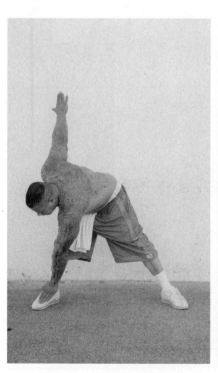 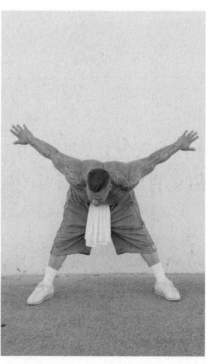 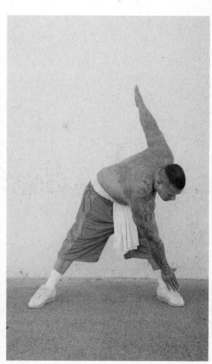

CHAPTER 5

Biceps and Triceps

These two muscle groups assist the back and chest in pulling and pushing movements, respectively. Triceps (located in the back of the upper arm) help the chest push people or things away while biceps (located in the front of the upper arm) help the back muscles pull people or things closer. Biceps also help lift and carry items around. If you've ever stood holding something heavy in your forearms, you likely know the feeling of soreness in your biceps later the same day.

Always be sure to work these smaller muscle groups after you've trained their larger counterparts. If you fatigue your biceps before working your back, your back workout will suffer. If you train your triceps before performing chest exercises your performance will also suffer. The routines provided by the inmates do an excellent job of making sure the large muscle groups are worked first, followed by the smaller assisting muscles.

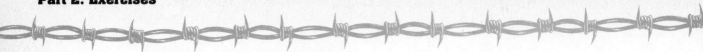

Back Arm Press

Your triceps will always be worked during push-ups, but in order to isolate and develop the back of your arm you're going to need to learn the back arm press. First, place your hands on an elevated surface (the higher the surface, the easier the exercise). With your hips placed higher in a slight pike position (a pike is like an inverted "V" in which your hips are the point of the letter and your hands and feet make up the ends), lower your body down with your elbows as the pivot joint. When you press up, the elbow will straighten and your body will rise back up to the original position.

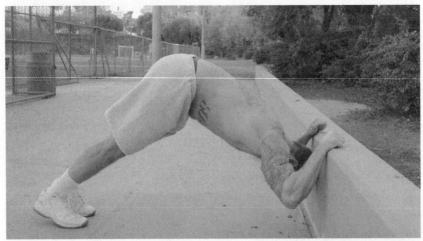

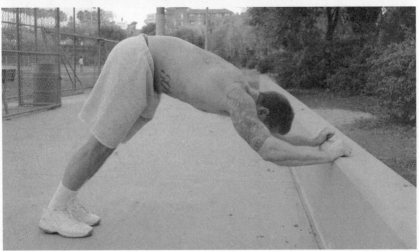

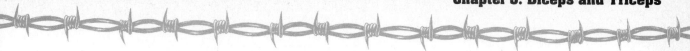

You can also perform a back arm press from the ground. Here, you can see the steeper angle of the body position (pike), which makes the exercise more difficult.

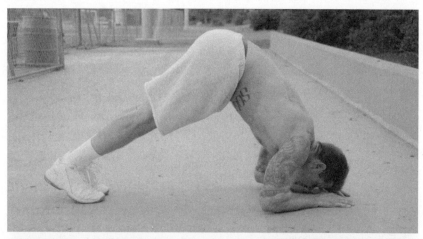

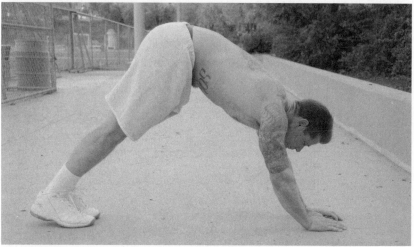

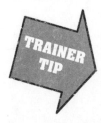

TRAINER TIP

Some inmates do back arm presses on the sink in their cell while others perform them on the toilet. You can try back arms wherever you like, making sure to lower the surface as you get stronger.

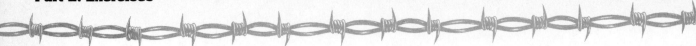

To mix up this exercise you can place your hands shoulder-width apart or closer together; experiment with hand position in order to learn what works best for you. Notice how the head lowers between the hands, forming a triangle with the two elbows.

⊘ CEASE AND DESIST

Avoid overhead triceps extensions and Skull Crushers, where you press dangerous amounts of weight directly over your head (moving just your forearms) using heavy barbells and dumbbells. A lot of dangerous gym equipment is necessary for these back of the arm exercises but back arm presses and the other tricep movements in this book will easily replace them.

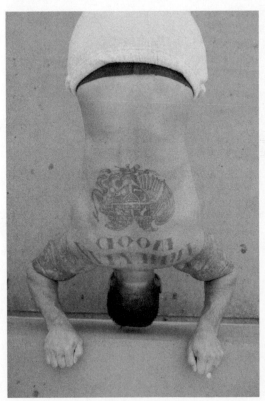
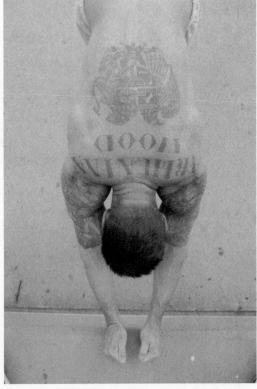

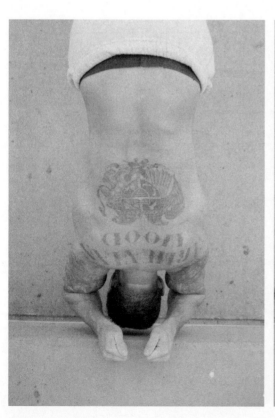 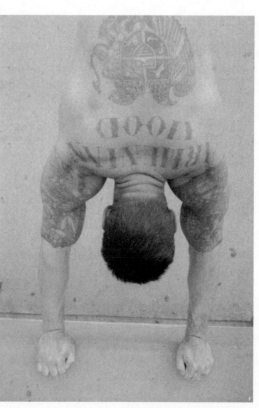

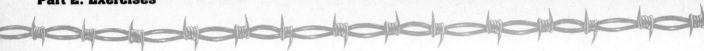

Bar Dips

Dips—which work your triceps, chest, and the front of the shoulder—are a deceptively hard exercise because (once again) you're moving all of your body weight with this multijoint movement. To perform this exercise, bend at the elbow while slowly lowering your body down toward the ground. Exhale as you press up, extending the arms and squeezing the tricep (the back of your arm) at the top of the movement. When lowering your body, it is safest to go down to the point at which your upper arm is parallel with the ground; going any lower puts undue strain on the shoulder. Keep your head up and your abs tight while performing this exercise. Remember that finding a place for dips is easy. You can use the seat of a chair, a knee-high ledge, your kitchen counter, the edge of your couch, a coffee table, and many other places to do dips.

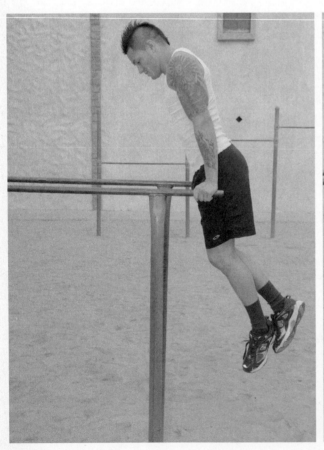 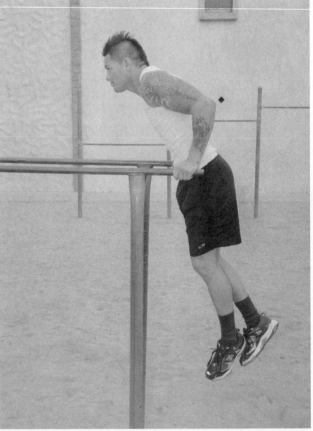

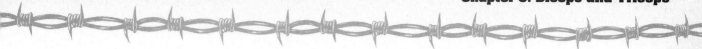

Many inmates wisely follow push-ups with this exercise in order to sculpt the back of the arm (triceps) and chest.

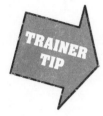

TRAINER TIP

During bar dips, keep your body vertical to put the focus on your triceps. Lean forward a bit during dips to transfer the exercise to your chest.

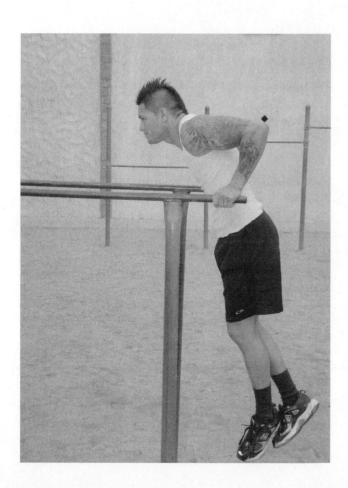

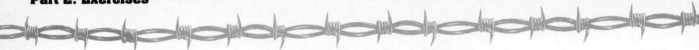

Diamond Dips (Bench Dips)

To perform a diamond dip, lower your body down toward the ground while keeping your feet on the ground and your hands close together on a low surface (bench, chair, couch, etc.). Push yourself up from the lowered position and squeeze the triceps (back of the arm) at the top of the movement.

Diamond dips allow you to focus more on the triceps because your hands are close together and your feet stay on the ground throughout the entire exercise. Make sure your hips drop straight down to keep the exercise focused on the back of the arm.

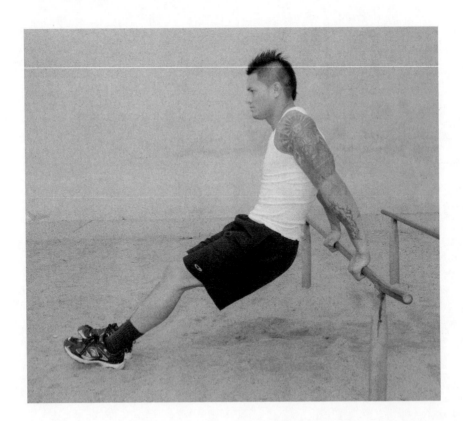

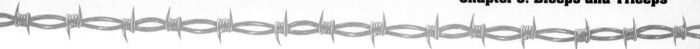

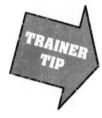TRAINER TIP

Extend your legs out to force your arms to do more work. If the exercise proves to be too easy, feel free to perform the exercise with one of your prison dumbbells resting on your thighs throughout each set for added resistance.

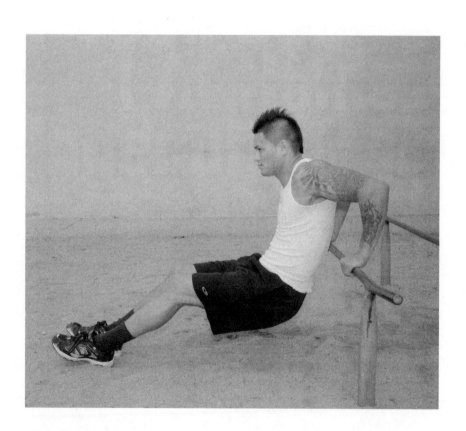

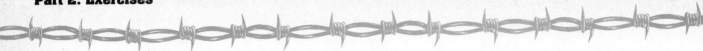

Curls

Hold the handles of your prison dumbbells with your palms facing up and your elbows held firmly against your sides as you lift up your hands, keeping your elbows locked in place. You'll feel the burn in your biceps and forearms right away.

Performing prison dumbbell curls with two hands puts the weight in the middle of your body, making it a challenge to keep the magazines from slamming into your abdomen. Regardless of how you decide to prevent the dumbbell from hurting you, be sure to keep your body supported with tightened abdominals and your shoulders held firmly back.

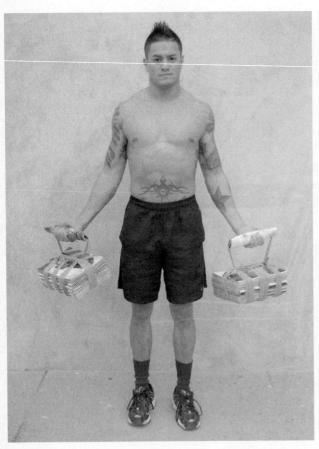
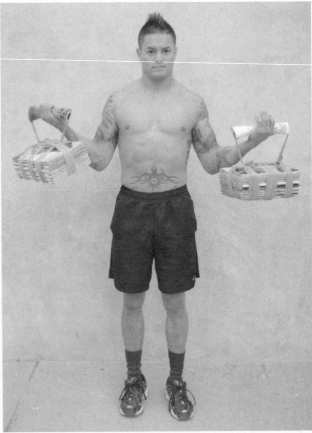

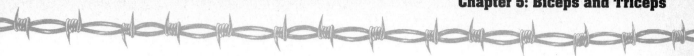

Concentration/"Peak" Curls

While seated or kneeling, position the back of your arm on the inside of your thigh. Proceed to curl the dumbbell up while keeping the back of your arm on your leg. Concentration curls force the biceps to do most of the work, since your leg is immobilized by your elbow. Few muscles assist the stationary arm in flexing the elbow, making this a favorite to give the biceps a higher "peak" and overall rounder look.

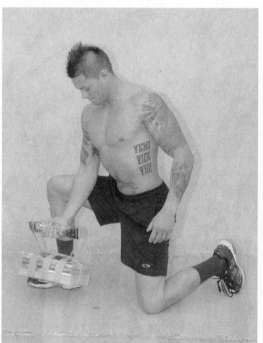 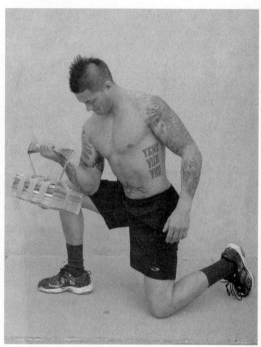

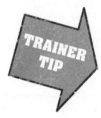

TRAINER TIP

Squeeze your biceps at the top of the movement to get maximum benefit from the exercise.

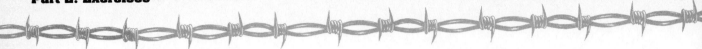

Reverse Curls

Your forearms get a workout from reverse curls. Simply hold your prison dumbbell with an overhand grip, stand with your feet shoulder width apart, and curl the weight up toward the top of the chest. Slowly lower the dumbbell and repeat.

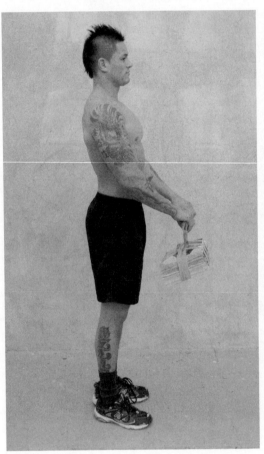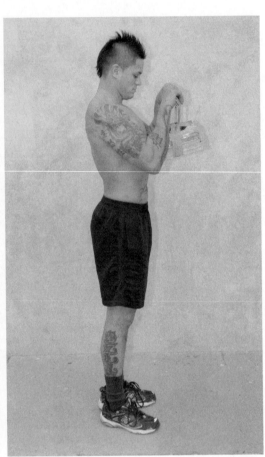

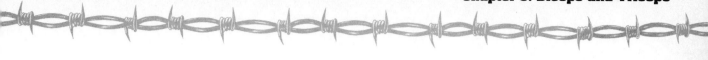

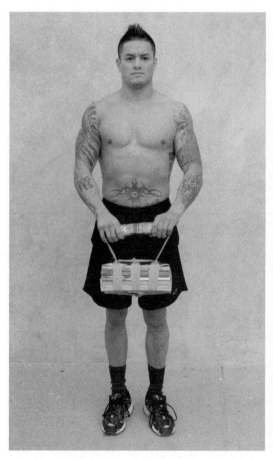
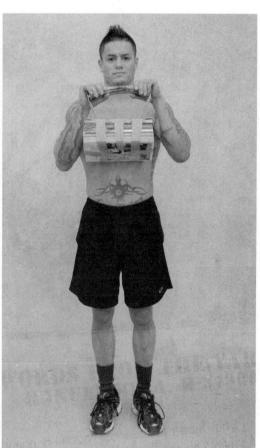

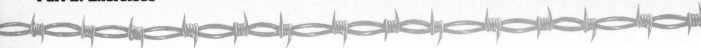

Hammer Curls

Hammer curls utilize a neutral grip; your palms are neither facing down nor up during a hammer curl. To help you do the exercise correctly, pretend you're raising your forearm to give a "thumbs-up" sign and make sure the thumb leads as the elbow flexes upward. This exercise targets the *brachioradialis*, the muscle that sits close to the elbow on the thumb side of the forearm.

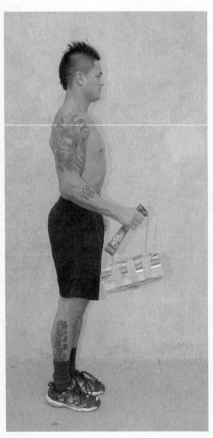 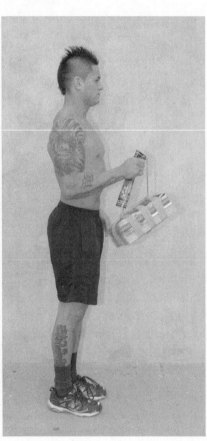 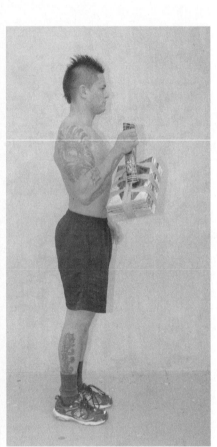

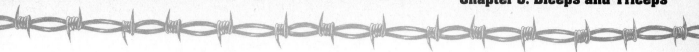

Wrist Curls and Reverse Wrist Curls

When seated on a chair or bench, place your forearms on your thigh so your hands hang over your knees. This position allows your wrists to flex and extend freely to perform the curls. Wrist curls are done with the palms facing up while holding the dumbbell, whereas reverse wrist curls are done with the palms facing down.

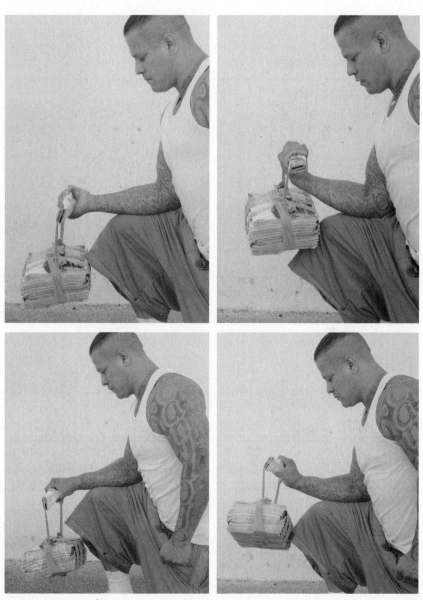

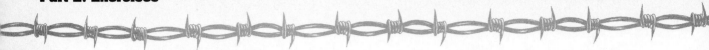

Kick-Outs

Also known as kick-backs, a kick-out is the final triceps exercise used to sculpt the back of the arm. Hold your prison dumbbells with your palms facing up and bend over with your back flat, and pull your elbows back to line up with your side. From this position extend your arms back and squeeze the triceps at the top of the movement for a great burn.

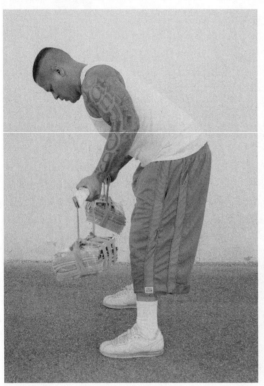 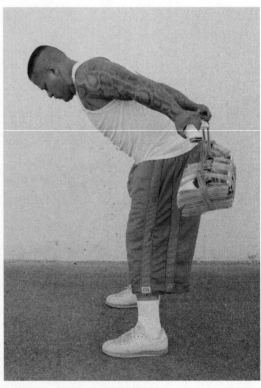

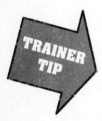

TRAINER TIP

Kick outs require a lighter weight than other exercises. Ten to fifteen pounds of resistance will likely be appropriate to complete a set.

CHAPTER 6

Abdominals

Before any of your other muscles contract, the abdominals lead the way to support your body. If your midsection isn't strong enough to support movement and extra weight, your body is going to find an alternate (and often dangerous) way to compensate for that lack of abdominal conditioning. When the abs don't do their fair share of work to support the spine when bending over, for example, the back and other muscle groups try to pick up the slack. That imbalance can lead to back injuries, hernias, and other painful conditions.

People often want a slim and lean stomach because it looks sexy—and great abs are one of the first things you think about when you think about a fit felon. But we encourage you to make that six-pack a secondary goal after you achieve a strong abdominal base. Strengthen your abs, tweak your diet, then strengthen the rest before you even start worrying about washboard abs. Wouldn't you rather remain injury-free and able to do all the things you enjoy than simply look good while unable to walk?

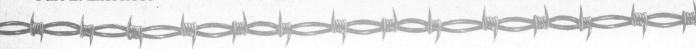

Crunches

To do a proper crunch, lift up your sternum (the bone in the middle of the chest) and forehead simultaneously in order to fully engage your rectus abdominus (the muscle that makes up the "six-pack"). Once you feel your shoulder blades come fully off the ground, carefully lower yourself back down before repeating. Keep your lower back pressed on the ground the entire time you do a crunch.

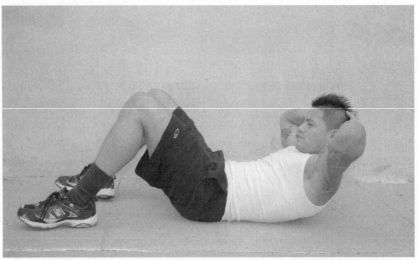

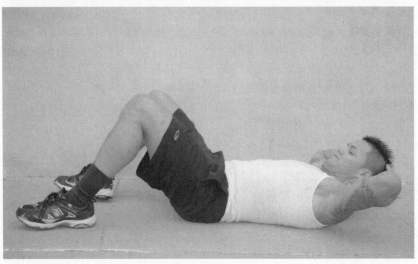

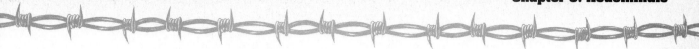

Reverse Crunches

To do a Reverse Crunch, first lift your hips and feet up off the ground, then curl your knees back toward your head in order to activate your abs. You then lower your hips down toward the ground first, before your feet tap the ground, finishing the exercise before you begin your next repetition.

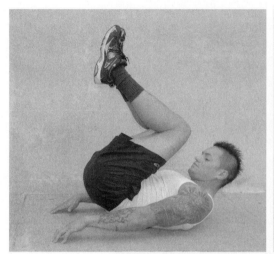
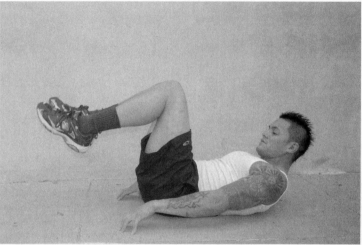

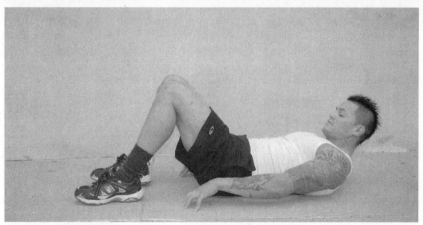

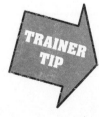

When doing a reverse crunch, keep your chin tucked down and visualize your knees coming up in an arc to hit your nose.

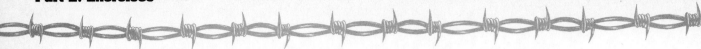

Oblique Crunch

When you do an oblique crunch you work your side abdominal muscles. These muscles (obliques) rotate the torso in twisting patterns. You'll lift your chest straight up doing this exercise, since your knees and hips will already be in a turned position. Keep your knees and ankles pulled together and touching the ground as you work through sets of oblique crunches. Always turn your legs to the other side and complete an equal number of reps.

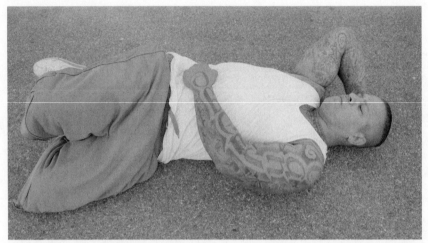

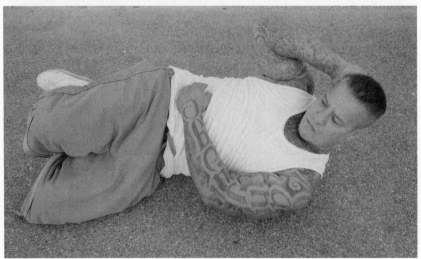

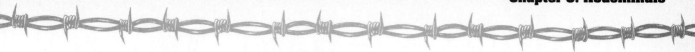

Cross-Leg Sit-Ups

With your left leg crossed over your right knee and your hands held behind your head, lift up your chest and ribs as you turn your right shoulder toward your left knee. Don't cheat by turning your elbow toward your knee. Keep the elbow back and focus on the turn and lift of the shoulder. This exercise works the sides of your abdominal wall.

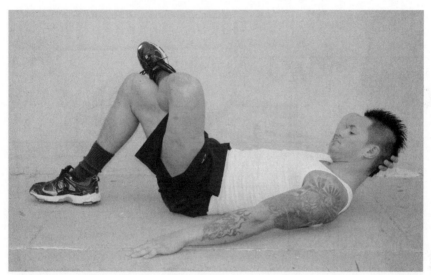

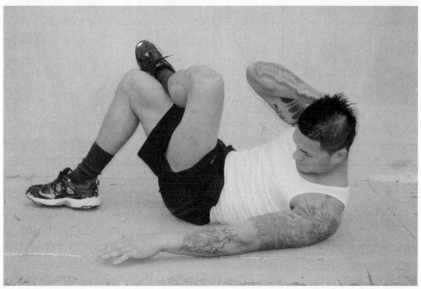

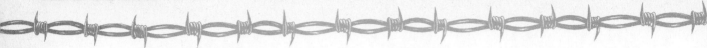

Leg Lifts

To perform leg lifts begin by lying down on a flat surface with your legs extended straight out. As you lift your legs into the air, pivot at the hip and slightly bend at the knee until your legs nearly make a 90-degree angle with your torso. Slowly lower your legs back to the ground before beginning your next repetition. Be sure to keep your abs tight and your lower back pressed on the ground while doing this exercise.

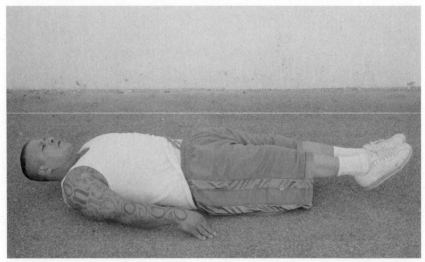

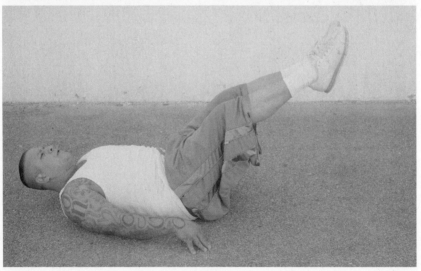

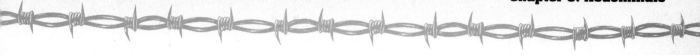

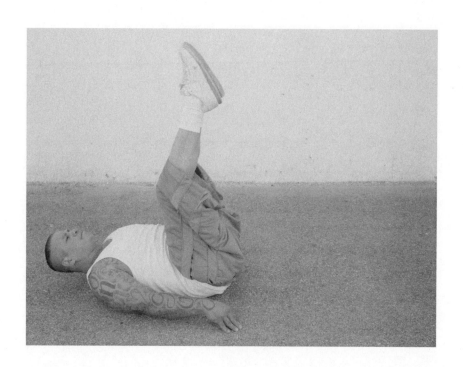

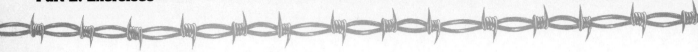

V-Ups

Arguably the most difficult of all the abdominal exercises done by the inmates is the V-up. This exercise requires both abdominal strength and flexibility in the back and hamstrings. While lying on the ground with your legs fully extended and your arms raised above your head, simultaneously lift up your legs and chest. Try to touch your toes with your fingers at the highest point possible.

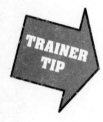

TRAINER TIP

The modified V-up is easier because you bend your knees as you come up. Reach for the space where your toes would be if your legs were straight.

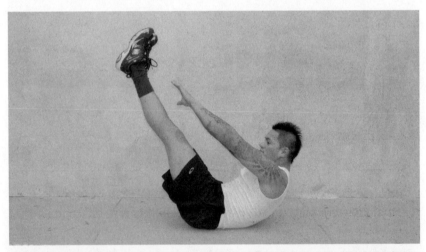

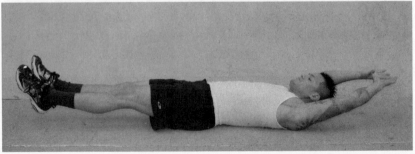

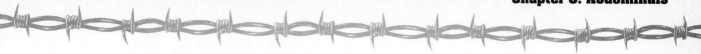

Side Busters

The side buster is a more advanced version of both the oblique crunch and the cross-leg sit-up. In addition to lifting the torso off the ground with your legs to one side, you now lift your legs as well.

With your left forearm and left hip on the ground, and your right hand behind your head, raise your right armpit up and forward. At the same time, lift your feet off the ground while keeping your ankles pressed together. You should feel a contraction on the right side of your abdomen. Switch sides and do the exercise again to complete a full rep.

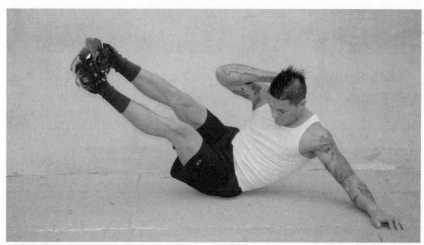

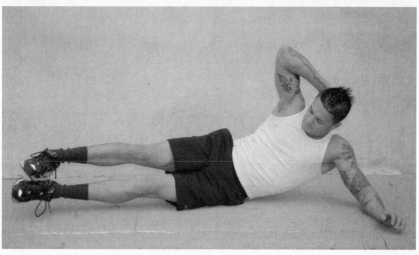

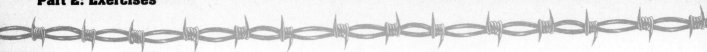

Hanging Oblique Leg Raises

The place that you do your pull-ups will double as the location for these hanging oblique leg raises. Hang from the bar with your arms straight and keep your knees and ankles together as you bring both of your legs up to the left and right of your body. As your abdominals and core get stronger you'll be able to complete this exercise without leaning back.

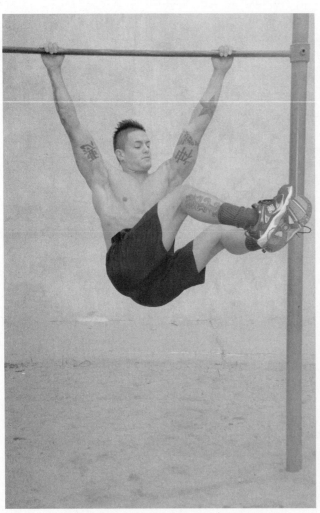
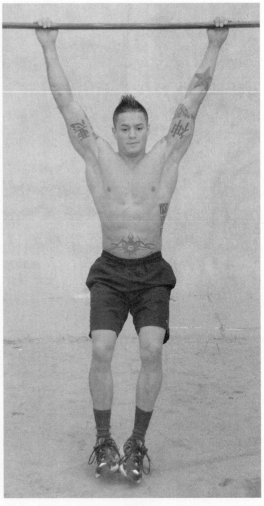

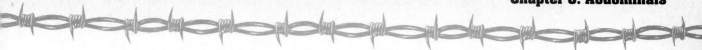

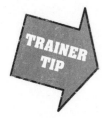

If you're lucky enough to have someone to work out with, have your partner stand behind you and support your lower back/hips with his or her hands. This support will keep your body from swinging and will prevent your shoulders from fatiguing too quickly so you can focus on your abdominal workout.

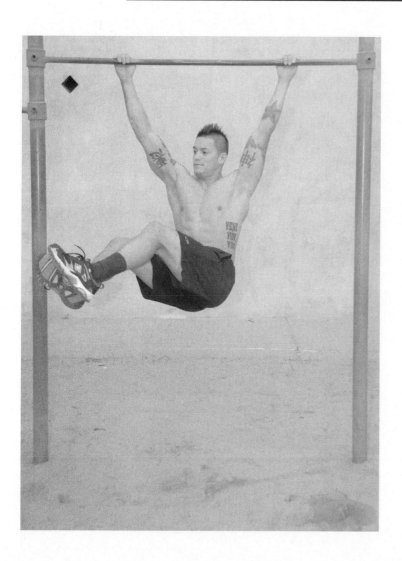

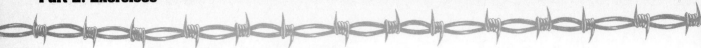

Standing Bicycle

A great way to work your abs without having to lie on the ground is the Standing Bicycle. With your feet about shoulder-width apart and hands behind your head, twist your right shoulder/torso to the left as you bring your left knee straight up. Return to the start position and reverse by twisting your left shoulder to the right as your bring your right knee straight up. One turn to each side completes one repetition.

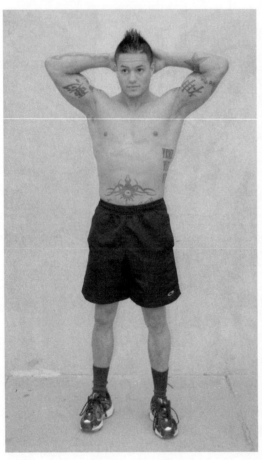
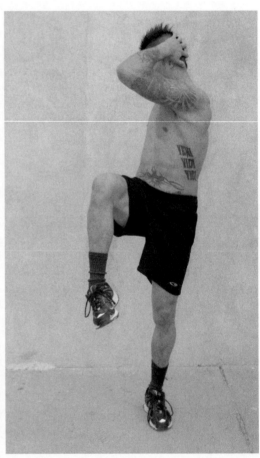

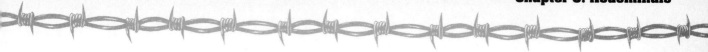

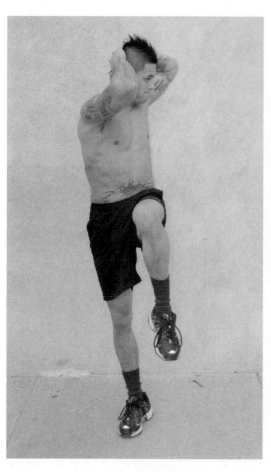
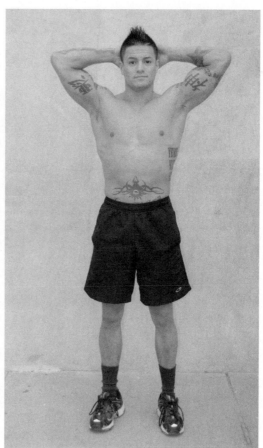

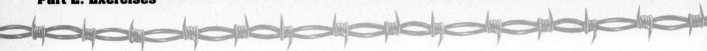

Mountain Climbers

This calisthenic exercise develops your aerobic capacity (what the inmates call "wind" or endurance) and challenges your core. To do Mountain Climbers, start by holding your body in a push-up position. Then start moving your legs as though you're running in a horizontal position with both of your hands on the ground. You've completed one repetition when each knee has come in toward the chest in succession.

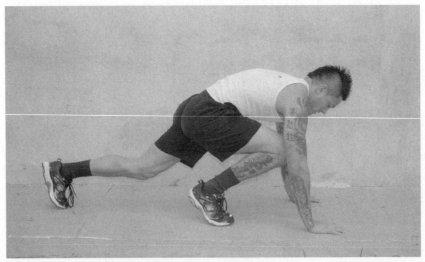

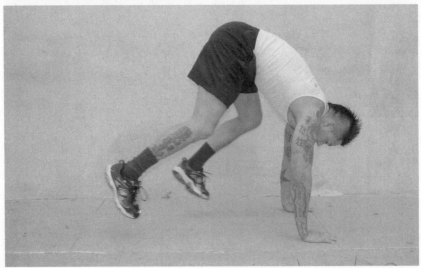

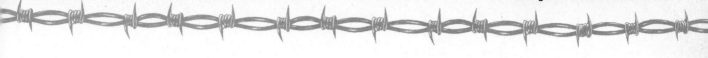

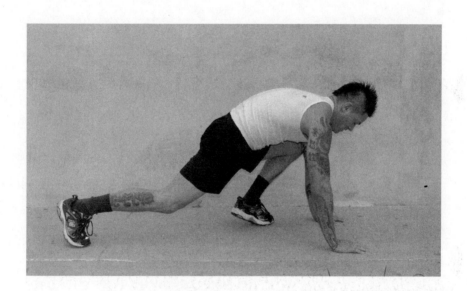

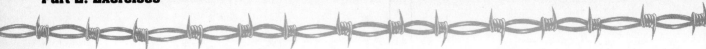

Knee Tucks

To do a knee tuck, start in a push-up position, then simply jump into a crouch position. Finish the rep by shooting your legs back out to their original push-up position. This exercise works your abdominals as well as your shoulder muscles.

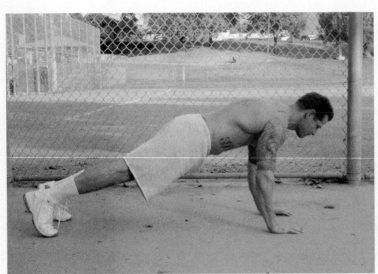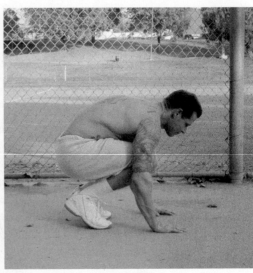

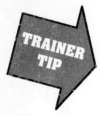

TRAINER TIP

Focus more on pulling in your knee than on hopping your feet forward. The knee-pull will help engage your abs and will reduce the amount of bouncing your hips will inevitably do while performing this exercise.

CHAPTER 7

Burpies

N o other exercise is as universally utilized in prison workouts as the burpie. And once you perform half a dozen
burpies you'll realize why so many inmates do them to
lose weight and stay in shape. This one exercise works many of your
muscle groups: You use your legs when you crouch down and stand
up; your chest, triceps, and front of your shoulders are taxed during
the push-up portion; and you use your abdominals to pull your legs
forward when you jump to the squat position.

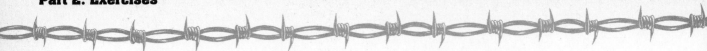

6-Count, 8-Count, and 10-Count Burpies

A burpie incorporates several different movements including one or more push-ups. For a 6-count burpie, from a standing position, crouch down and place your hands on the ground. From there, shoot your legs back into a push-up position. Perform a push-up, hop back to the crouch, and stand again. In an 8-count burpie, you do two push-ups, and in a 10-count, you do three push-ups.

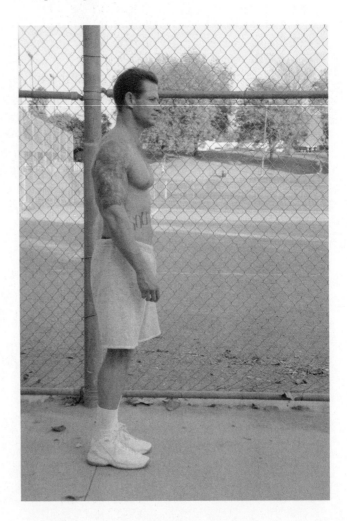

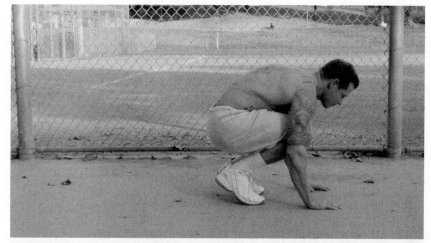

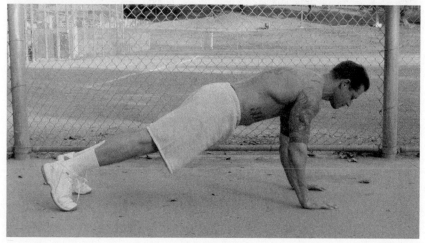

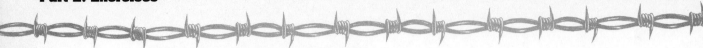

Navy SEAL Burpie

For the Navy SEAL Burpie, start as you would any burpie by crouching down, placing your hands on the ground outside of your feet, and shooting your legs back to a push-up position. Then, as you move away from the ground during the first push-up, bring a knee in toward your chest between your arms. The knee that just came in to your chest straightens and goes back to the ground as you're performing the next push-up. Bring the opposite leg into the chest as you're completing the second push-up. As the second leg returns to the ground, begin a third push-up without any knee movement before you spring your legs back up to a crouch position and stand to complete the burpie. The action of bringing the knees in adds to the difficulty of the exercise and incorporates more of an abdominal component to the exercise.

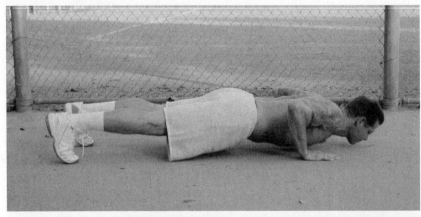

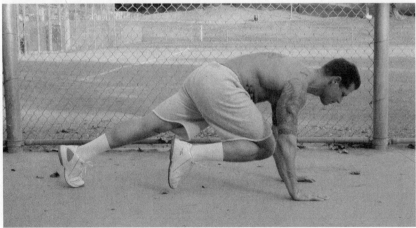

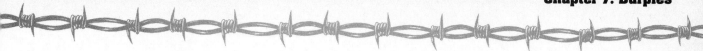

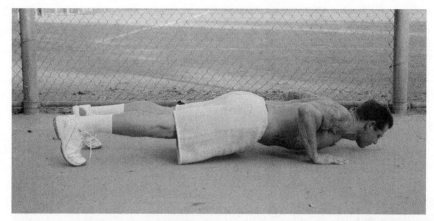

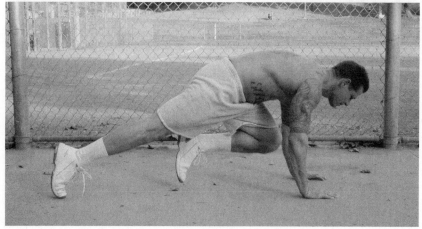

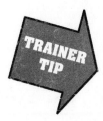

Feel free to try any of the different types of push-ups in the middle of your burpies. If an inmate's routine calls for 100 burpies, we suggest you try 20 burpies with regular push-ups, 20 with diamond push-ups, 20 with wide push-ups, 20 with staggered hands (right hand closest to the body), and finish with 20 more staggered-hand push-ups (left hand closest to the body). You'll have to widen your stance for diamond push-ups, but aside from that minor adjustment you won't have to do anything other than count accurately and change the push-up once it's time to switch to another variety.

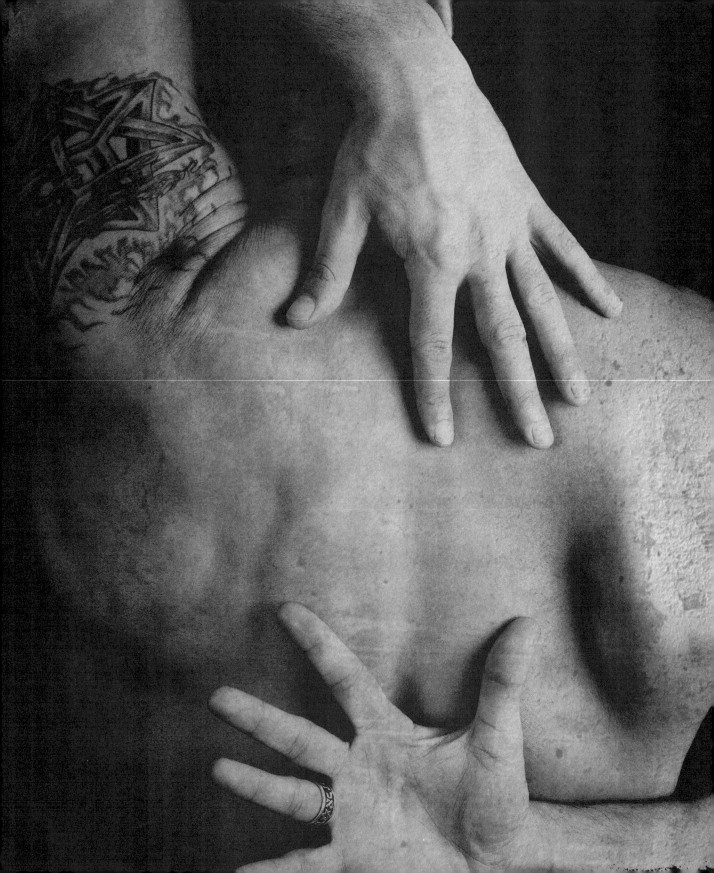

PART 3
Stretches

Stretching is an important and often overlooked element of exercise that needs to be done after workouts. When you work a muscle group such as your legs, you tighten the muscles from all the contractions performed throughout squats, lunges, step-ups, etc. In order to keep your legs from staying tight and restricting movement, you need to stretch the muscles you've trained (the thighs, hips, butt, back of the legs). The same is true when you work your back, chest, shoulders, and arms. Always stretch the muscle groups that you've just trained.

Contrary to popular belief, static stretching (a stretch that is held for at least 20 seconds) before a workout is not a good idea. The stretch will only inhibit your muscles' abilities to contract and produce force. A pre-workout stretch will also make joints more lax, opening up the opportunity for injury since maintaining form during exercise will prove more difficult.

Stretches need to be held for a minimum of 20 seconds, three times. So, for example, if you stretch your right hamstring followed by your left, you'll have to stretch each two more times. That will add up to roughly three minutes of hamstring stretching. That time is a small price to pay compared to the time you might lose from rehabbing after you pull a muscle.

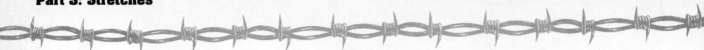

Cross-Arm Shoulder/Back Stretch

By simply holding your arm across your chest and holding on to it with the opposite arm you stretch the middle part of your back (trapezius, rhomboid) along with your shoulders (deltoid). Stand up straight and hold your core tight while doing any standing stretch. Perform this stretch after shoulder work.

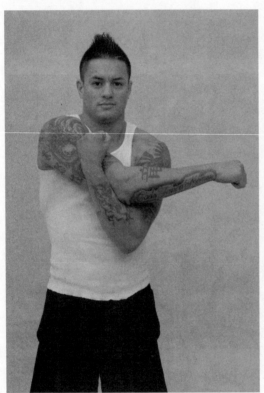
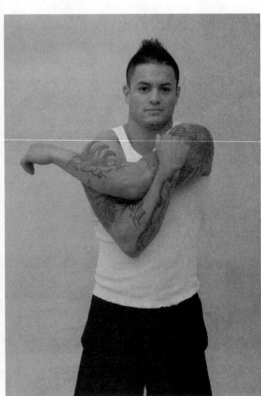

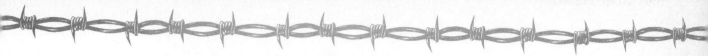

Standing Toe Touch

Stand with your feet hip-width or closer and reach down to touch your toes. This stretch lengthens the hamstring group as well as the lower and middle part of the back. You can bend your knees slightly if the stretch is too much to handle at first. Always do this stretch after a leg workout.

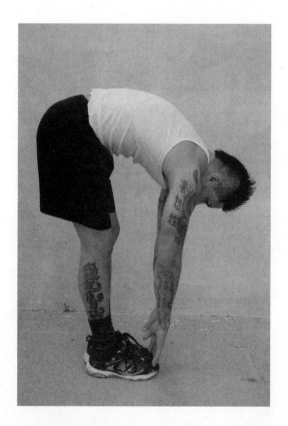

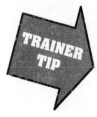

TRAINER TIP

Go to *www.bmi-calculator.net* to learn your current body mass index. Normal BMI ranges from 18.5 to 24.9.

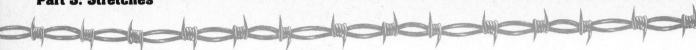

Wide-Leg Reach

With your legs held twice as wide as your shoulders, reach down to each foot and hold the stretch for at least 20 seconds. You can also stretch by reaching toward the center of your stance, below your pelvis. Stretching at different angles is a great way to target different muscles. When doing a wide-leg reach you target your hamstrings and back along with your outer and inner thigh (abductors and adductors). This stretch is another must after leg workouts.

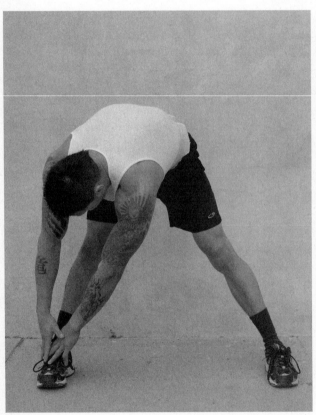
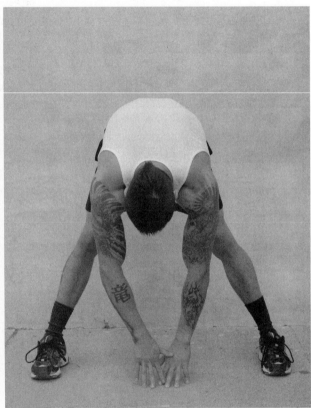

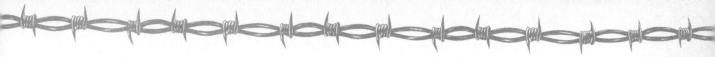

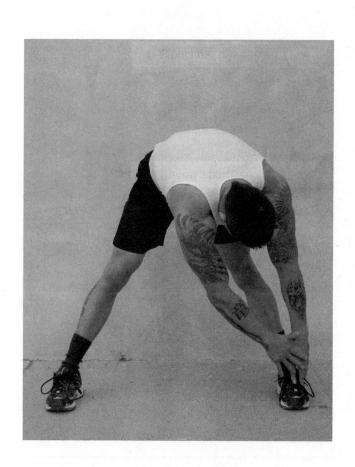

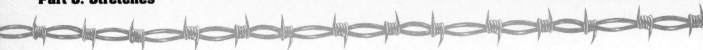

Standing Quadriceps Stretch

There's nothing novel about this stretch, but it is great to help keep your thigh muscles loose, preventing knee problems. From a standing position, pull your right foot up and back toward your rear end while keeping your knees under your hips. Be sure to switch and stretch your left foot.

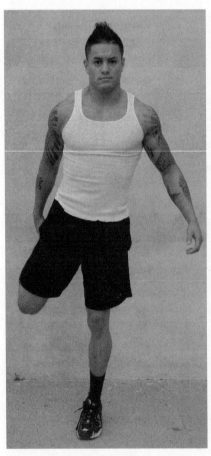 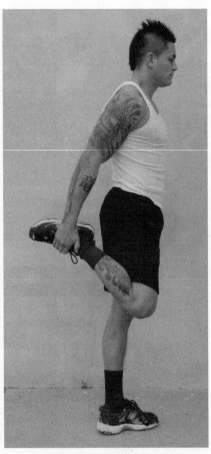

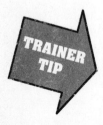

To intensify the stretch move the knee of the leg being stretched further back behind the hips/pelvis, lengthening the quadriceps and hip flexors (muscles that move your upper leg forward and up, as you walk, run, step up, etc.) even more intensely.

Standing Knee Pull

Stand and pull your knee into your chest. Hold your shoulders back and keep your core tight. This stretch is an excellent way to target your rear end and upper part of your hamstring. This stretch is also a good test of your balance. Be sure to alternate knees to stretch both side of your hips and hamstrings.

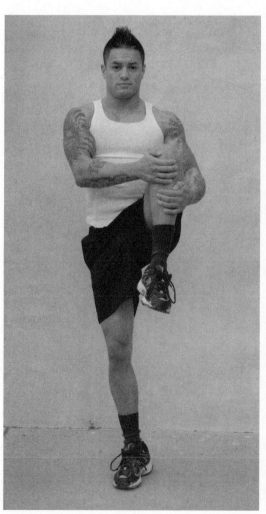 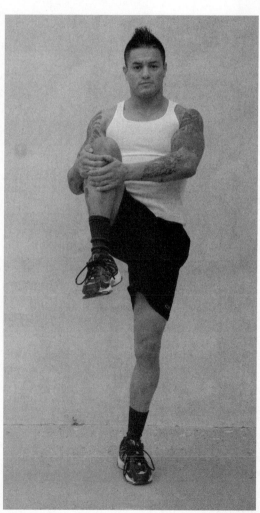

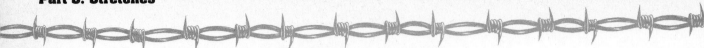

Overhead Triceps Stretch

After a workout full of dips or back arm presses, be sure to complete this stretch. Hold your arm straight up over your head and let your hand drop below your neck. Use your nonstretching arm to simultaneously pull your elbow back and push your forearm down to intensify the stretch.

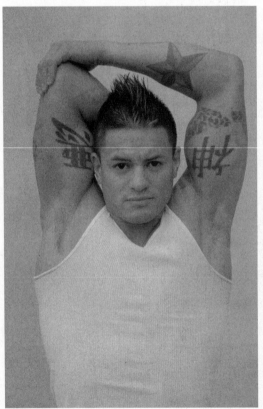 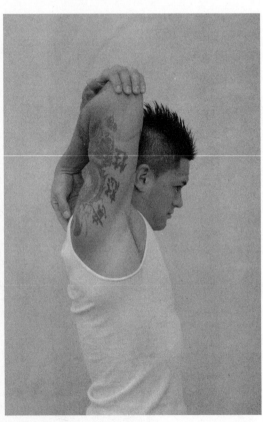

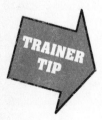

TRAINER TIP

It's never too late to start an exercise program. Losing weight has immediate benefits, so exercise will improve your health whether you are thirty years old and fifty pounds overweight or fifty years old and ten pounds overweight.

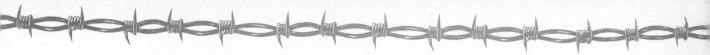

Hip Flexor Stretch

This stretch does a great job of lengthening the quadriceps (front of the thigh) and iliacus/psoas major, the muscles that flex your hips and allow you to kick your leg up. If you sit at a desk all day your hip muscles are contracted for hours. If you then exercise with movements similar to running or lunging you are actively flexing those muscles. Use this stretch to counter the effects of all that hip flexing in order to help ease tightness in your hips and lower back. This stretch also is great if you like to run because it targets muscles that tighten from running.

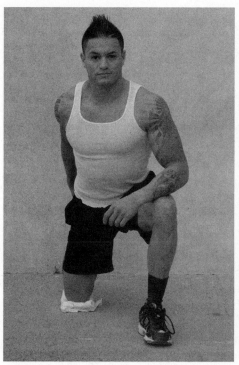 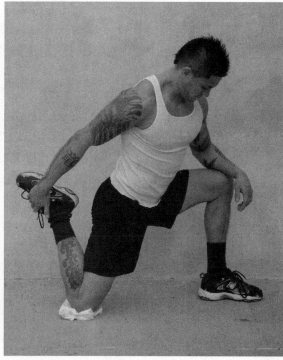

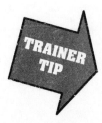

TRAINER TIP

The more you lean into the position and pull your heel toward your butt, the more you will feel this stretch. Keep your shoulders, hips, and your front foot all facing squarely in the same direction.

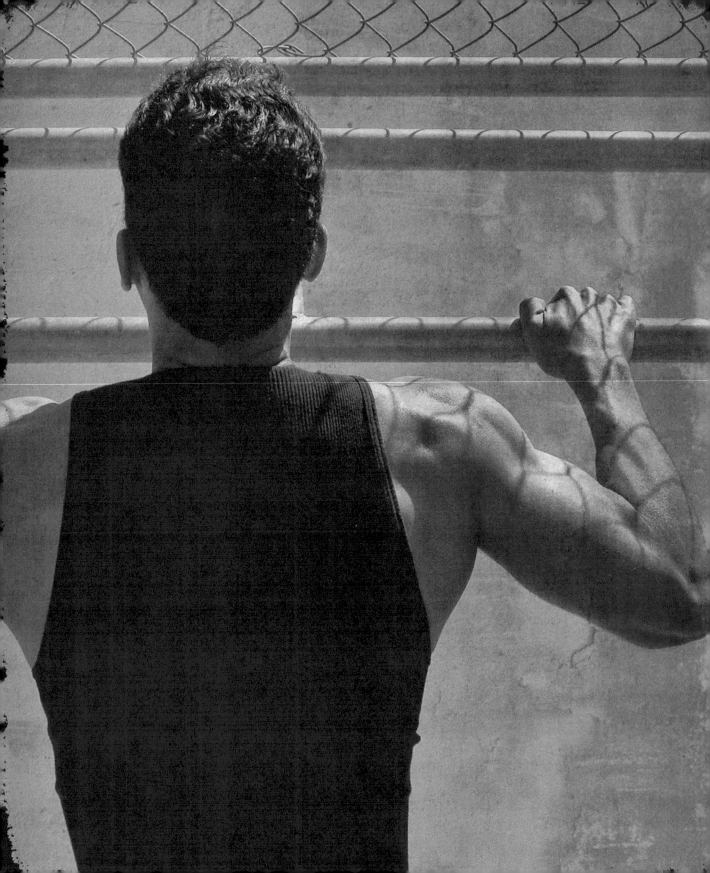

PART 4
Inmate Workout Routines

If you want the hard body of an inmate, then the best thing you can do is follow an actual inmate's workout routine. We've given you the exercises and stretches that you need to get it done, and here, nine inmates (whom you'll learn more about on the rap sheet that begins each chapter) take you through the detailed workouts that have increased both their muscle mass and endurance and made them a force to be reckoned with in the yard.

As you get started it's important for you to keep in mind that these workouts are not easy. The inmates have to perform a high volume of repetitions when they exercise because they don't have access to weights. In spite of this, they are very well conditioned and it's likely that you won't be able to perform as many repetitions as they do when you first begin to follow their programs. The simple trick will be for you to start with fewer reps and then build your way up as your endurance increases.

As you work your way through the workouts you'll notice that there are exercises marked with numbers followed by letters (1a., 1b., 1c., etc.); this designation means that these exercises are supersets and/or circuits that are done in succession, without stopping. You can take a break between each set.

Example Routine

EXERCISE	SETS	REPS
1a. Push-ups	10	20
1b. Squats	10	20

In this example you would perform twenty push-ups immediately followed by twenty squats. You would then take your rest period after the squats, before your next superset starts with push-ups. Here you're doing ten supersets total.

So now that you know what's in store, it's time for you to either put up or shut up and start working out—like a felon.

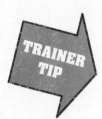

TRAINER TIP

Time how long it takes you to complete all of your routines and record the results. Challenge yourself by trying to finish each routine in progressively less time.

CHAPTER 8

J. Pinedo [K-14865]

Inmate Rap Sheet

Name: J. Pinedo	**CDCR#:** K-14865
Age: 34	**Height:** 5'9"
Weight before prison: 215 pounds	
Weight after beginning prison workout plan: 185 pounds	
Length of incarceration: Sentenced 30 to Life	
Time served: 15 years	
About the Inmate: Mr. Pinedo was our go-to guy when it came to correspondence. He did a great job of coordinating our efforts within the prison walls to collect the exercise programs of other inmates. As an inmate, Mr. Pinedo knows the other men who work out and was able to recruit people he felt could offer us good routines and sensible advice.	

DAY 1

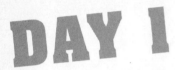

K-14865 starts his routine by working out his back and chest. Remember that pull-ups work your back along with your biceps and forearms, push-ups work your chest and triceps, and dips work your triceps, along with your chest and shoulders. The running burns extra calories during this inmate's workout and likely does a great job of keeping his heart rate elevated. The increased heart rate in this routine keeps your muscles from cooling down when they're not being worked during exercise, preventing injury.

Start today off with a 5–7 minute warm-up with jogging and stretching.

Endurance and Strength Circuits

EXERCISE	SETS	REPS
1a. Pull-ups (grip varied)	10	15
1b. Dips (grip varied)	10	20
1c. Push-ups (grip varied)	10	20
1d. Run ¼ mile at 75% of max	10	1

* Rest 60–90 seconds between sets.

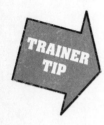

TRAINER TIP

Many of the inmate routines include running. If you can't run, walk at a brisk pace. Use the odometer in your car to map out a few routes in your neighborhood. Rotate the routes in your routine to avoid boredom. Incorporate a hill or two if you can to make your workout really challenging. Plan your route to pass things you enjoy seeing, like a beautiful view, neighbors who say hello but don't chat (you don't want them stopping you and interrupting your workout), or a pretty woman/handsome man.

DAY 2

Do a 5–7 minute warm-up with jogging and stretching.

Legs and Core

EXERCISE	SETS	REPS
1a. Calf raises	3	100
1b. Squats	3	30
1c. Lunges	3	30

* Rest 45 seconds between sets.

EXERCISE	SETS	REPS
2a. Calf raises	5	100
2b. Jump-squats	5	20
2c. Plyometric lunges	5	20

* Rest 1 minute between sets.

EXERCISE	SETS	REPS
3a. Pistol squats (each leg)	3	10
3b. Step-ups	3	50

* Rest 45 seconds between sets.

EXERCISE	SETS	REPS
4a. Hanging leg raises	10	20
4b. Crunches	10	50

* Rest 45 seconds between sets.

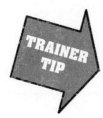

TRAINER TIP

Unilateral (one-sided) exercises, such as lunges and pistol squats, help address any strength imbalances in your legs. Everybody is stronger on one side of his or her body—if you're left-handed, your left arm is almost always stronger (your dominant side), and the opposite is true for right-handed individuals. If you exercise properly by doing an equal number of repetitions and an equal amount of weight on each side of your body (arms and legs), you'll reduce those imbalances to a nearly imperceptible level.

DAY 3

Day 3 is a day of rest, but this doesn't mean that Pinedo lies around all day. He's very athletic and plays sports on the days he doesn't actively train— and to keep yourself fit, you should too.

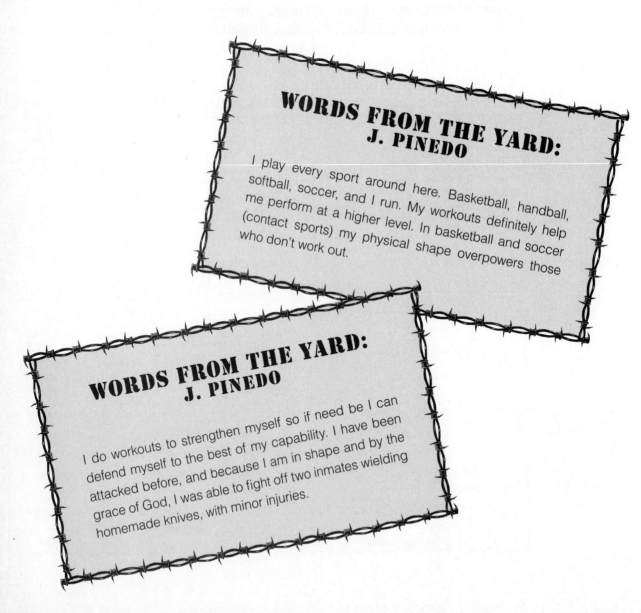

WORDS FROM THE YARD:
J. PINEDO

I play every sport around here. Basketball, handball, softball, soccer, and I run. My workouts definitely help me perform at a higher level. In basketball and soccer (contact sports) my physical shape overpowers those who don't work out.

WORDS FROM THE YARD:
J. PINEDO

I do workouts to strengthen myself so if need be I can defend myself to the best of my capability. I have been attacked before, and because I am in shape and by the grace of God, I was able to fight off two inmates wielding homemade knives, with minor injuries.

DAY 4

Today the focus is on the back with this simple (but not easy) pull-up routine. Remember, you'll work forearms and biceps quite a bit when you use an underhand grip. If you can't do sets of 20, max out every set.

Start today off with a 5–7 minute warm-up that includes jogging and stretching, and cool down with stretching once you've completed the routine.

Strength Training: Back

PULL-UPS	SETS	REPS
1. Full motion w/pause at top (overhand)	4	20
2. Close-grip (overhand grip)	4	20
3. Behind neck (overhand grip)	4	20
4. Close-grip (underhand grip)	4	20
5. Wide grip (underhand grip)	4	20

* Rest 2–3 minutes between sets.

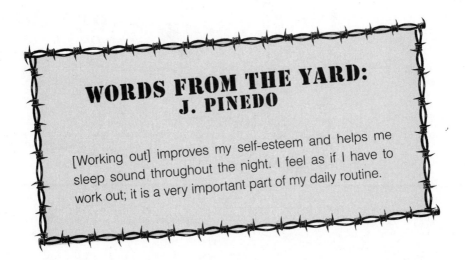

WORDS FROM THE YARD:
J. PINEDO

[Working out] improves my self-esteem and helps me sleep sound throughout the night. I feel as if I have to work out; it is a very important part of my daily routine.

DAY 5

Today's routine is another chest and triceps workout with a heavy focus on triceps (the back of the arm). Days 2 through 4 don't work the chest, making day 5 the perfect time to go back to push-ups and back arm presses.

Start today with a 5–7 minute warm-up that includes jogging and stretching.

Strength Training: Triceps and Chest

EXERCISE	SETS	REPS
1a. Dips	20	To failure
1b. Push-ups (grips varied w/ pause, don't fully extend to keep muscles tense)	20	To failure
2. Back arm presses	20	To failure

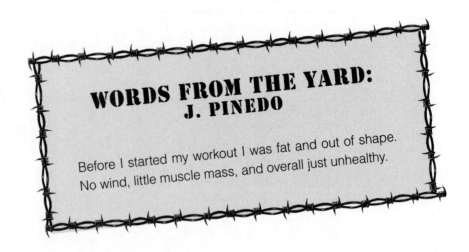

WORDS FROM THE YARD: J. PINEDO

Before I started my workout I was fat and out of shape. No wind, little muscle mass, and overall just unhealthy.

DAY 6

Remember that endurance workouts are the name of the game when it comes to survival in California State Prison. The high volume of repetitions in today's workout will make you lean and mean. We've given you a few options for Day 6, so pick your poison.

Start today with a 5–7 minute warm-up that includes jogging and stretching.

Strength: Option 1

EXERCISE	SETS	REPS
1a. Push-ups	20	To failure
1b. Dips	20	To failure
1c. Pull-ups (varied grips)	20	To failure
Run sprints for 20 minutes (all-out max for 45 seconds, rest 60, repeat)		

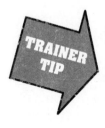

Sprinting is an excellent way to boost natural levels of GH (growth hormone), which in turn speeds tissue (muscle, tendon, ligament) recovery and helps build lean muscle.

Strength: Option 2

EXERCISE	SETS	REPS
1. Regular push-ups	1	To failure
2. Wide push-ups	1	To failure
3. Diamond push-ups	1	To failure
4. Decline push-ups	1	To failure
5. Staggered-hand push-ups	1	To failure
6. Back arm press	10	20
7. Handstand press	10	To failure

Rest 1–1½ minutes between sets.

This day 6 option is a great total-body routine using body weight for resistance while incorporating functional exercises in the form of push-ups and squats. Establish a steady pace and you'll find that this routine is a great aerobic workout and isn't tedious like running on a treadmill. Start with a 5–7 minute warm-up with jogging and stretching.

Endurance and Cardio: Option 1

EXERCISE	SETS	REPS
1a. Plyometric push-ups	20	25
1b. Jump squats	20	25
1c. Jumping jacks	20	25

* There should be little or no rest between sets.

Finish with 15 minutes of intense jump-rope

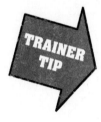

If you feel you're not ready for plyometric exercise or think you're too old for explosive movements, simply reduce jump squats to regular squats, plyometric push-ups to push-ups, and so on.

Cardio Option

Remember that a steady pace will help you get through this routine; it's a marathon, not a sprint.

Endurance and Cardio: Option 2 (Full-Body Workout)

EXERCISE	SETS	REPS
1. Jumping jacks	3	100
2. Push-ups	3	25
3. Squats	3	50
4. 6-count burpies	3	25
5. Standing bicycles	3	50
6. Push-ups	3	25
7. Lunges (Lunges are done on both legs. Make sure you do the same number of repetitions on both sides.)	3	50
8. 8-count burpies	3	25
9. Shoulder rotations (arms fully extended)	3	50
10. Push-ups	3	25
11. Calf raises	3	50
12. 10-count burpies	3	25

* Don't rest for more than 45 seconds between exercises.

CHAPTER 9

Jeffrey "Bandit" Goldstein [T-35745]

Inmate Rap Sheet

Name: Jeffrey Goldstein	**CDCR#:** T-35745
Age: 29	**Height:** Unknown
Weight before prison: Unknown	
Weight after beginning prison workout plan: 200 pounds	
Length of incarceration: Sentenced to 23 years	
Time served: 11 years	

About the Inmate: The routines we received from Bandit take him one hour to complete. These workouts look like a huge amount of exercise, but truly you'll be repeating just a few exercises with progressively fewer repetitions, which will help you build endurance and strength. Again, if the volume of exercise is too much (and it may be) reduce the number of reps to a fraction of what Bandit performs and build your way up.

As you look at Bandit's workout routine, you'll notice that he makes a common mistake among gym-going males—he doesn't work his legs enough. How many men have you seen in gyms with well-developed upper-bodies and skinny legs? A lot, right? Too often men forget that increased muscle mass in the legs will boost testosterone levels, making it possible (and a lot easier) to maintain and further develop the upper body. However, even though Bandit doesn't spend enough time on his legs, he does do a great job of working his chest, shoulders, and back and, luckily, there are several workouts from other inmates in this book that train the lower-half of the body just as thoroughly as Bandit does his upper body. Don't be afraid to combine the various inmate workout routines to find what works best for you.

Note: When Bandit does his early-morning routine, he takes things up a notch by not resting between the various exercises. Not only does that make his workout more time efficient, it also keeps his heart rate elevated, making the routine a great form of aerobic conditioning.

MONDAY, WEDNESDAY, FRIDAY

1,000 Push-Ups, 1,000 Calf Raises, and 400 Squats (4:30 A.M.–5:30 A.M. in Cell)

EXERCISE	SETS	REPS
1a. Push-ups	5	50
1b. Calf raises	5	50
2a. Push-ups	5	30
2b. Calf raises	5	50
3a. Push-ups	5	25
3b. Calf raises	5	50
4a. Diamond push-ups	5	20
4b. Calf raises	5	50
5a. Diamond push-ups	5	15
5b. Squats	5	20
6a. Decline push-ups	5	25
6b. Squats	5	20
7a. Decline push-ups	5	20
7b. Squats	5	20
8a. Decline push-ups	5	15
8b. Squats	5	20

Dips, Decline Push-Ups, and Back Arm Presses (2:00 P.M.–3:00 P.M. in Recreation Yard)

EXERCISE	SETS	REPS
1a. Shoulder-width diamond dips	10	10
1b. Decline push-ups	10	15–20
2a. Chest-width diamond dips	5	10
2b. Back arm presses	5	20–25

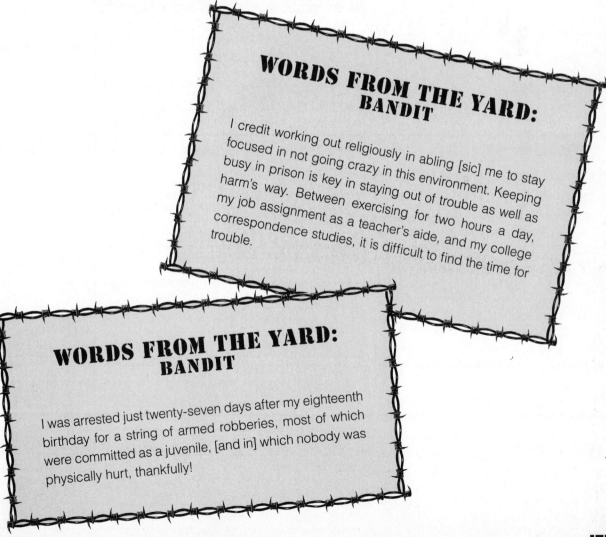

WORDS FROM THE YARD: BANDIT

I credit working out religiously in abling [sic] me to stay focused in not going crazy in this environment. Keeping busy in prison is key in staying out of trouble as well as harm's way. Between exercising for two hours a day, my job assignment as a teacher's aide, and my college correspondence studies, it is difficult to find the time for trouble.

WORDS FROM THE YARD: BANDIT

I was arrested just twenty-seven days after my eighteenth birthday for a string of armed robberies, most of which were committed as a juvenile, [and in] which nobody was physically hurt, thankfully!

TUESDAY, THURSDAY, SATURDAY

(4:30 A.M.–5:30 A.M. IN CELL)

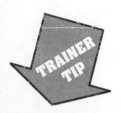

Remember to work your way up in terms of intensity (weight) and volume (number of repetitions). If you can do all the repetitions with 20 pounds, you should then think about increasing the weight to 25 pounds. When you find a weight that matches your limits, you can then start adding volume to your routine. Increase intensity and volume in increments of 5.

Prison Dumbbell Workout (40–45 Pounds)

EXERCISE	SETS	REPS
1a. Curls (shoulder-width)	5	25
1b. Cherry Pickers	5	20
2a. Curls (shoulder-width)	5	20
2b. Cherry Pickers	5	20
3a. Curls (shoulder-width)	5	15
3b. Cherry Pickers	5	20
4a. Curls (chest-width)	5	20
4b. Cherry Pickers	5	20
5a. Curls (chest-width)	5	20
5b. Cherry Pickers	5	20
6a. Curls (chest-width)	5	15
6b. Cherry Pickers	5	20
7a. Upright rows	5	15
7b. Chain Breakers	5	20
8a. Upright rows	5	10
8b. Chain Breakers	5	20
9a. Upright rows	5	5
9b. Chain Breakers	5	20
10a. Shrugs	5	40
10b. Arm rotations (forward and backward)	5	20
11a. Shrugs	5	30
11b. Arm rotations (forward and backward)	5	20

TUESDAY, THURSDAY, SATURDAY
(2:00 P.M.–3:00 P.M. IN RECREATIONAL YARD)

Once you finish the exercises in the following table, take a 1-mile jog at a regular pace.

Pull-Ups

TYPE OF PULL-UP	SETS	REPS
"As wide as possible"	5	8–10
Shoulder-width	5	8–10
Overhand behind neck	5	5–8

SUNDAY
(2:00 P.M.–3:00 P.M. IN RECREATIONAL YARD)

- ✘ 1-mile jog (fast-paced)
- ✘ 100 burpies (6-count)
- ✘ ¼-mile walking lunges

CHAPTER 10

Dennis James Baltierra [E-57085]

Inmate Rap Sheet

Name: Dennis James Baltierra	CDCR#: E-57085
Age: 45	Height: Unknown
Weight before prison: 165 pounds	
Weight after beginning workout plan: 183 pounds	
Length of incarceration: Unknown	
Time served: 9 years	

About the Inmate: As the oldest inmate to submit a workout routine, Dennis adjusts his workouts according to the limits of his body. You'll notice in the Week 1 and Week 3 overview (Dennis submitted a month-long workout routine) that Dennis performs his "push weight" exercises twice and the "pull-weight" exercises once. He then reverses the routine and does "pull-weight" exercises twice (in Week 2 and Week 4) and the "push-weight" exercises once. That reversal is a smart way to make sure muscle groups receive equal amounts of rest and exercise during a given program.

Because of his age, Dennis also rests on Saturdays and Sundays. He may be active with sports on the weekend, but he refrains from any strenuous activity to let his body recover properly. If you're getting up there in years, Dennis's workout will likely be a great fit for you.

WEEK 1 AND WEEK 3 OVERVIEW

Monday: Push-weight exercises

Tuesday: Calisthenics, martial arts, and shadow-boxing exercise with stretches

Wednesday: Pull-weight exercises

Thursday: Calisthenics, shadow-boxing, martial arts defense, and stretch exercise

Friday: Push-weight exercise

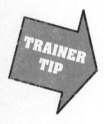

TRAINER TIP

Exercise releases endorphins, which reduce stress and give you a general feeling of calm and relaxation. Feeling stressed? Work out!

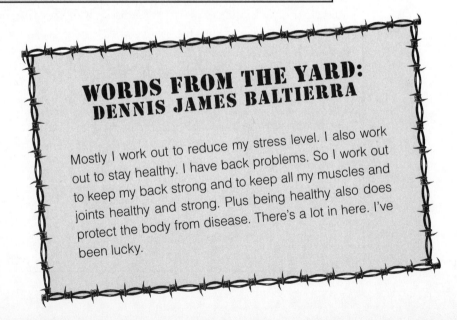

WORDS FROM THE YARD: DENNIS JAMES BALTIERRA

Mostly I work out to reduce my stress level. I also work out to stay healthy. I have back problems. So I work out to keep my back strong and to keep all my muscles and joints healthy and strong. Plus being healthy also does protect the body from disease. There's a lot in here. I've been lucky.

WEEK 2 AND WEEK 4 OVERVIEW

Monday: Pull-weight exercises

Tuesday: Calisthenics, martial art shadow boxing exercise with stretches

Wednesday: Push-weight exercise

Thursday: Calisthenics, martial art shadow boxing exercise with stretches

Friday: Pull-weight exercise (You'll notice that Dennis makes no mention of doing pull-ups during his "pull-weight" days. His age and a previous shoulder injury likely prevent him from doing pull-ups.)

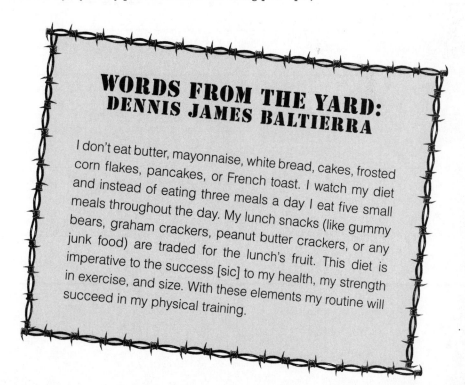

WORDS FROM THE YARD: DENNIS JAMES BALTIERRA

I don't eat butter, mayonnaise, white bread, cakes, frosted corn flakes, pancakes, or French toast. I watch my diet and instead of eating three meals a day I eat five small meals throughout the day. My lunch snacks (like gummy bears, graham crackers, peanut butter crackers, or any junk food) are traded for the lunch's fruit. This diet is imperative to the success [sic] to my health, my strength in exercise, and size. With these elements my routine will succeed in my physical training.

Push-Weight Exercise Routine

EXERCISE	SETS	REPS
1. Lateral raise with a book (start with a small book and work yourself up to a large dictionary or encyclopedia)	10	15
2. Curl and press	10	To failure (as many as possible in 30 seconds)
3. Overhead press #1	3 with 25-lb dumbbell	20
4. Overhead press #2	3 with 35-lb dumbbell	15
5. Overhead press #3	4 with 45-lb dumbbell	To failure
6a. Push-ups	10	20
6b. Squats	10	25

* Perform this workout at an easy pace with no rest between sets.

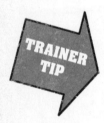

TRAINER TIP

Just because Dennis doesn't do pull-ups doesn't mean you can't. Feel free to add them into your routine if you think your body can take it.

Pull-Weight Exercise Routine (with 45-pound, 35-pound, and 25-pound prison dumbbells)

EXERCISE	SETS	REPS
1. Curls	3	20
2 Single-arm curls	4	6–8
3. Curls	3	To failure
4. Lawn Mowers (also known as a dumbbell row)	3 with 35-lb dumbbell	20–30
	3 with 45-lb dumbbell	10–20
	4 with 25-lb dumbbell	To failure

* Take a 30-second rest between every set.

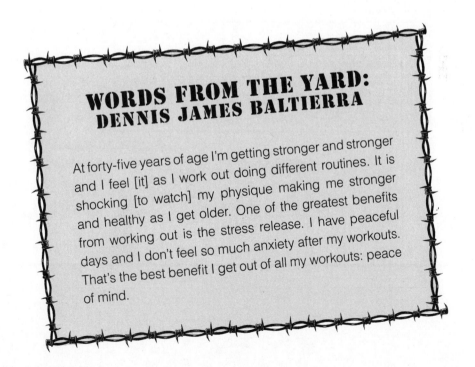

WORDS FROM THE YARD: DENNIS JAMES BALTIERRA

At forty-five years of age I'm getting stronger and stronger and I feel [it] as I work out doing different routines. It is shocking [to watch] my physique making me stronger and healthy as I get older. One of the greatest benefits from working out is the stress release. I have peaceful days and I don't feel so much anxiety after my workouts. That's the best benefit I get out of all my workouts: peace of mind.

Dennis performs the following circuit three times, as fast as he can. Remember, for a routine to be a circuit, you have to perform the next exercise on the list immediately after you finish the one before it. With that said, the following eleven exercises should be done back-to-back before you rest for a minute or two. You will then begin the circuit again until you've completed it three times.

Calisthenics Circuit

EXERCISE	SETS	REPS
1. Push-ups	3	25
2. Jumping jacks	3	50
3. Squats	3	50
4. Atomic sit-ups	3	20
5. Mountain climbers	3	75
6. Push-ups	3	25
7. Jumping jacks	3	50
8. Standing bicycles	3	50
9. Atomic sit-ups	3	15
10. Push-ups	3	20
11. Squats	3	50

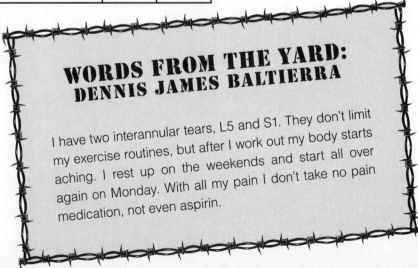

WORDS FROM THE YARD:
DENNIS JAMES BALTIERRA

I have two interannular tears, L5 and S1. They don't limit my exercise routines, but after I work out my body starts aching. I rest up on the weekends and start all over again on Monday. With all my pain I don't take no pain medication, not even aspirin.

CHAPTER 11

Alejandro Perez

[V-43776]

Inmate Rap Sheet

Name: Alejandro Perez	CDCR#: V-43776
Age: 28	Height: Unknown
Weight before prison: 110 pounds	
Weight after beginning prison workout plan: 150 pounds	
Length of incarceration: Unknown	
Time served: 11 years	

About the Inmate: When Alejandro gave us his workouts he reminded us that on some days inmates are not allowed out of their cells due to mandatory prison lockdowns that administrators say are for the safety of inmates and prison guards. When prohibited from leaving their cells inmates have no access to pull-up bars, dip bars, running tracks, or the rest of the prison yard to play sports. On such days inmates alter their workouts; such cell workouts translate easily to programs that can be performed outside of prison.

Do you travel for business? Have you ever been stuck in a hotel room because you either don't have access to transportation or you're in an unfamiliar city and aren't sure where to go? Don't just sit around watching basic cable; this is the perfect opportunity to complete one of the workouts provided by Alejandro. The only items you'll need will be the hotel bed (to put your feet up on for incline push-ups), your packed suitcase (for curls and upright rows), and enough floor space to shoot your legs out into a push-up position for burpies. All hotel rooms have enough space and furniture to finish a cell workout and, as an added bonus, these workouts don't take very long.

Before you get started, please note that Alejandro does the following warm-up before all of his workouts:

- ✖ Stretches (10–15 minutes)
- ✖ Cross-arm shoulder stretch
- ✖ Overhead triceps stretch
- ✖ Toe-touch
- ✖ Standing quad stretch
- ✖ Jumping-jacks (50)

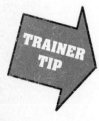

TRAINER TIP

Be strict with the amount of time you take between sets during a cell workout. Consistent breaks will make it easier for you to notice results because you'll be ready to start with less time between sets as you continue the workouts week after week.

MONDAY, WEDNESDAY, FRIDAY

Cell Workout

EXERCISE	SETS	REPS
1. 10-count burpies	1	50
2a. Regular push-ups	6	25
2b. Squats	6	20
3a. Wide push-ups	6	25
3b. Calf raises	6	25
4a. Incline push-ups	6	25
4b. Squats	6	20
5a. Diamond push-ups	6	25
5b. Calf raises	6	30
6. Oblique crunches	7	15
7. Reverse crunches	7	15
8. Modified V-ups	7	15

TUESDAY, THURSDAY

Cell Workout

EXERCISE	SETS	REPS
1. 10-count burpies	1	100
2a. Single-arm book curls	10	15
2b. Upright rows	10	15
2c. Back arms	10	20

* Take a 25-second rest between the previous sets.

EXERCISE	SETS	REPS
3. Oblique raised-leg crunches (take a 15-second rest between sets)	7	15
4. Reverse crunches (take a 15-second rest between sets)	7	15
5. Modified V-ups (take a 15 second rest between sets)	7	15

MONDAY, WEDNESDAY, FRIDAY

Yard Workout

EXERCISE	SETS	REPS
1. * Wide-grip pull-ups	5	10
2. * Close-grip pull-ups	5	10
3a. Dips	10	10
3b. Regular push-ups	10	25
3c. Back arms	10	20
4. Regular push-ups	5	25
5. Wide push-ups	5	25
6a. Hanging oblique knee raise	8	5
6b. Hanging knee raise	8	10
6c. Straight-arm oblique knee raise	8	10

Take a 30-second rest between each set

* Note: Alejandro does wide-grip pull-ups with his hands held twice as wide as his shoulders. He holds his body at the top of the pull-up for seven seconds before lowering himself down slowly. He has his hands touching (all the way together) for close-grip pull-ups.

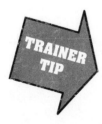
TRAINER TIP

Delayed onset muscle soreness, a.k.a. "DOMS," will be present during your first few weeks of working out but will decrease as you continue training.

TUESDAY, THURSDAY

Run 1 mile before starting the following routine.

Yard Workout

EXERCISE	SETS	REPS
1. Behind-the-back pull-ups	5	10
2. Close-grip pull-ups	5	10
3a. Behind-the-back pull-ups	5	10
3b. Incline push-ups	5	25
4a. Diamond push-ups	5	25
5a. Alternating oblique knee raise	8	5
5b. Hanging knee raise	8	10
5c. Alternating oblique knee raise	8	10

* Take a 30-second rest between each set and/or superset.

CHAPTER 12

Manuel Meza
[H-37966]

Inmate Rap Sheet

Name: Manuel Meza	**CDCR#:** H-37966
Age: 35	**Height:** Unknown
Weight before prison: 193 pounds	
Weight after beginning prison workout plan: 170 pounds	
Length of incarceration: Unknown	
Time served: 11 years	

About the Inmate: Manuel's routines are intense upper-body workouts. His arm routine isolates your biceps and triceps, which leads to excellent strength development and an increase in muscle mass. His chest routine is equally challenging given the intensity of the "celly" push-ups and the volume of regular push-ups that follow. The pyramid burpie portion of his Wednesday workout is nothing short of exhausting. You can count on developing your aerobic system, chest endurance, and leg strength upon completing Manuel's workouts.

MONDAY, THURSDAY

Arm Routine

EXERCISE	SETS	REPS
1a. Concentration curl	4	10
1b. Back arm press	4	30
2a. Standing dumbbell curl*	4	6–8
2b. Back arm presses (as slow as possible)	4	15
* 3-second raise and 4-second release		
3a. Hammer curls*	4	6–8
3b. Back arm press	4	To failure
* 2-second raise and 3-second release		
4a. Reverse curls	4	20
4b. Hammer curls	4	6–8
5a. Upright row	4	15–20
5b. Lateral arm raises (no weight)	4	30–50
6a. Front raise (palms down)	4	4–6
6b. Arm rotations (each direction)	4	75

* Rest 1 minute between supersets.

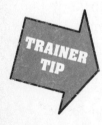

TRAINER TIP

To strengthen your hands/grip try one of Manuel's favorite exercises, handball squeezes. For this exercise, just find a ball the size of an apple and squeeze it for four sets of ten repetitions.

TUESDAY, FRIDAY

Chest Routine

EXERCISE	SETS	REPS
1. Celly/partner push-ups	5	6–8
2a. Dumbbell single-arm flies	4–5	8
2b. Push-ups	4–5	25
3a. Push-ups	4	25
3b. Jumping jacks	4	50
4a. Push-ups	4	10
4b. Mountain climbers	4	10
5. Push-ups with alternating leg kicks	4	15–20

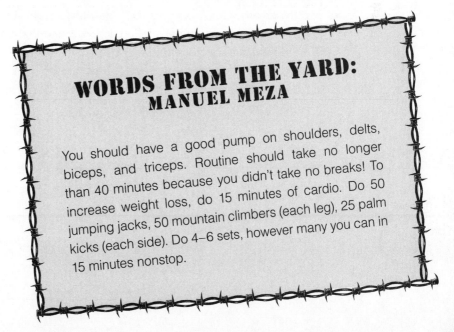

WORDS FROM THE YARD:
MANUEL MEZA

You should have a good pump on shoulders, delts, biceps, and triceps. Routine should take no longer than 40 minutes because you didn't take no breaks! To increase weight loss, do 15 minutes of cardio. Do 50 jumping jacks, 50 mountain climbers (each leg), 25 palm kicks (each side). Do 4–6 sets, however many you can in 15 minutes nonstop.

WEDNESDAY
Endurance and Power

On Wednesdays Manuel performs four exercises that really develop his aerobic conditioning. Clearly he knows that aerobic/cardiovascular fitness is important since he incorporates burpies. His other routines are excellent for strength and muscular development of the chest, triceps, shoulders, and biceps. He doesn't write about doing pull-ups, but if you were to add them definitely do so at the beginning of the Monday/Thursday routine. Otherwise you'll exhaust your arms with curls, making pull-ups close to impossible.

If you do the math associated with Manuel's progressive/pyramid scheme you'll notice that the exercises he recommends add up to 20 burpies, which in turn add up to 210 push-ups and 210 squats. All the energy expended doing this up-and-down routine will really build your aerobic capacity, as well as strengthen your legs and sculpt your chest.

- ✖ Handstand push-ups (10 reps)
- ✖ 10 push-ups into 10 mountain climbers (repeat 5 times)
- ✖ Knee-tucks (40 reps)
- ✖ Progressive/pyramid burpies: Do one burpie with a push-up at the bottom. Complete two squats before starting the next burpie. On the next burpie you will do 2 push-ups. Complete 3 squats before starting the next burpies. The next burpie will include 3 push-ups. This progression continues until you perform 20 squats and 20 push-ups with the last burpie.

CHAPTER 13

Tom McDonald
[T-79116]

Inmate Rap Sheet

Name: Tom McDonald	**CDCR#:** T-79116
Age: 33	**Height:** 5'8"
Weight before prison: 198 pounds	
Weight after beginning prison workout plan: 151 pounds	
Length of incarceration: Sentenced to 33 years	
Time served: 8 years, 9 months	

About the Inmate: Throughout Tom McDonald's workout you'll see a lot of aerobic exercises, which this inmate does because he easily puts on weight. Each day McDonald power-walks ten laps, which adds up to 2.5 additional miles of aerobic exercise. You'll notice that Tom doesn't exercise on Mondays—maybe it's an equally stressful day of the week on the inside just as it is on the outside. Regardless, you need to give your body time to recover, so taking at least one day a week off from exercise is absolutely necessary.

TUESDAY

This Tuesday workout is done with supersets—each set of curls is followed immediately by a set of back arm presses. Rest 1 minute between supersets.

Arms

EXERCISE	SETS	REPS
1. Biceps curls (wide-grip, shoulder-width, close-grip)	5–8 (1 set with each grip)	30 (10 of each grip mentioned)
2. Back arm press	5–8	50

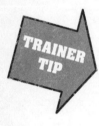

TRAINER TIP

Use a tape measure to see where you lose and/or gain size on your body. Measuring is a great way to track your progress and keep you motivated.

WEDNESDAY

Chest and Back

EXERCISE	SETS	REPS
1. 6-count burpies	1	500
2. Pull-ups/chin-ups*	10	10–12

* In between each set of pull-ups or chin-ups, power-walk ¼ mile.

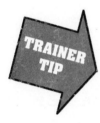

TRAINER TIP

How many people do you know who have injured themselves because they tried to "work through" pain and ignored the warning signs their body gave them? Those people hurt themselves and immediately regret their mistake of trying to forge ahead. Any injury takes weeks and often months to heal, but preventative rest and recovery takes only a few days. Listen to your body and you'll reduce the frequency and severity of injuries you incur.

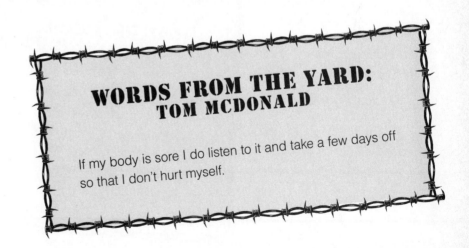

WORDS FROM THE YARD:
TOM MCDONALD

If my body is sore I do listen to it and take a few days off so that I don't hurt myself.

THURSDAY

Chest and Triceps

EXERCISE	SETS	REPS
1. Side busters (each side)	3	100
2. Crunches	3	100
3. Lower-back extensions	3	100

* Above performed any time before 12 noon.

4. 5-mile run		
5. Push-ups	10	50
6. Dips	10	15

* In between each set of the two exercises (push-ups and dips), power-walk a ¼-mile lap.

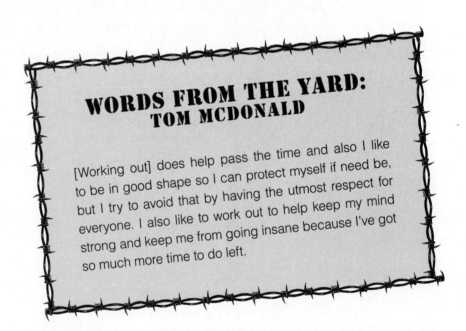

WORDS FROM THE YARD:
TOM MCDONALD

[Working out] does help pass the time and also I like to be in good shape so I can protect myself if need be, but I try to avoid that by having the utmost respect for everyone. I also like to work out to help keep my mind strong and keep me from going insane because I've got so much more time to do left.

FRIDAY

Cardio and Core

EXERCISE	SETS	REPS
1. Side busters (each side)	3	100
2. Crunches	3	100
3. Lower-back extensions	3	100

* Above performed any time before 12 noon

4. 4-mile run		
5. 6-Count Burpies	1	500

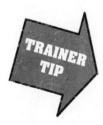

TRAINER TIP

Listen to your body, but don't get lazy. There's a fine line there between pushing yourself toward an injury and using the excuse of injury prevention to avoid exercise. Only you will know where you stand.

SATURDAY

Tom performs this workout right after breakfast. The energy he gets from his first meal seems to be a great boost for his workout. Some people might feel nauseated exercising after eating, so feel free to perform this routine before you eat if you prefer.

Abs and Cardio

EXERCISE	SETS	REPS
1a. Side busters (right side)	3	100
1b. Crunches	3	100
1c. Side busters (left side)	3	100

* In between each set of abs, do 100 lower-back extensions.

2. 3-mile run		
3. 6-count burpies	1	500

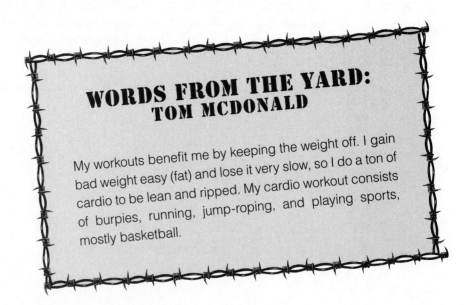

WORDS FROM THE YARD:
TOM MCDONALD

My workouts benefit me by keeping the weight off. I gain bad weight easy (fat) and lose it very slow, so I do a ton of cardio to be lean and ripped. My cardio workout consists of burpies, running, jump-roping, and playing sports, mostly basketball.

SUNDAY

Tom performs this workout right after breakfast. The energy he gets from his first meal seems to be a great boost for his workout. Some people might feel nauseated if they exercise after eating, so feel free to perform this routine before you eat if you prefer.

Abs

EXERCISE	SETS	REPS
1a. Side busters (right side)	3	100
1b. Crunches	3	100
1c. Side busters (left side)	3	100

* In between each set of abs, do 100 lower-back extensions.

Legs

EXERCISE	SETS	REPS
Squats	10	100

* In between each set of squats, power-walk ¼-mile lap.

Note: The last 15 reps of each set is jump-squat.

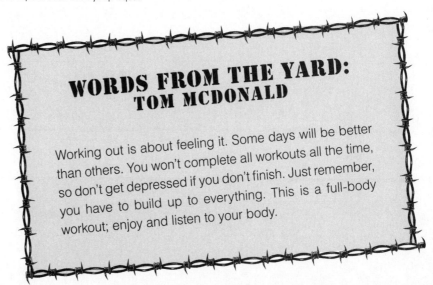

WORDS FROM THE YARD:
TOM MCDONALD

Working out is about feeling it. Some days will be better than others. You won't complete all workouts all the time, so don't get depressed if you don't finish. Just remember, you have to build up to everything. This is a full-body workout; enjoy and listen to your body.

CHAPTER 14

Anthony Sarmiento
[T-44463]

Inmate Rap Sheet

Name: Anthony Sarmiento	**CDCR#:** T-44463
Age: 30	**Height:** Unknown
Weight before prison: 155 pounds	
Weight after beginning prison workout plan: 168 pounds	
Length of incarceration: Unknown	
Time served: 10 years	

About the Inmate: When you look at this inmate's workout routine, you'll notice that Anthony works out only three times a week, but he stays active in other ways. He enjoys playing sports while in prison, which makes staying healthy and fit that much easier. If you can find an activity that you enjoy doing, you'll be fit and healthy without trying—and without overtraining or losing interest, as often happens with people who get bored with their workout routines.

MONDAY AND FRIDAY

Upper Body (No Shoulders)

EXERCISE	SETS	REPS
1. Jumping jacks	1	50
2a. Back arm presses	10	10
2b. Curls	10	10
2c. Push-ups	10	30

* Rest for 20 seconds between every set of the three exercises.

EXERCISE	SETS	REPS
3. 1-mile jog		
4a. Behind-neck pull-ups	10	8
4b. Bar dips	10	25

* Rest for 20 seconds after each set of dips.

EXERCISE	SETS	REPS
5a. Pull-ups (underhand grip)	10	8
5b. Bench dips	10	25

* Rest for 10 seconds after each set of dips.

EXERCISE	SETS	REPS
6. 1½-mile jog		

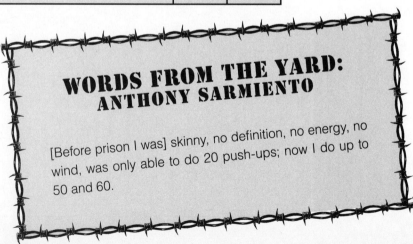

WORDS FROM THE YARD:
ANTHONY SARMIENTO

[Before prison I was] skinny, no definition, no energy, no wind, was only able to do 20 push-ups; now I do up to 50 and 60.

TUESDAY

EXERCISE

Handball and basketball

WORDS FROM THE YARD: ANTHONY SARMIENTO

[Working out] makes me feel good about myself . . . gives me self-confidence. It's also a big stress reliever. When I feel a little stressed or depressed I work out.

WORDS FROM THE YARD: ANTHONY SARMIENTO

I've tried to do the Monday–Friday routine, but I found it made me always tired, weak, and bored. The every-other-day routine I saw the most results in, and I felt more energy. The thing that keeps me in shape the most is I think sports. You got to be really active and full of energy, and you'll notice once you're done your whole body will be tired.

WEDNESDAY

Legs, Shoulders, and Abs

EXERCISE	SETS	REPS
1. Jumping jacks	1	50
2. Squats (with weight)	5	25
3. Jump squats	10	15–20
4. Lunges	10	25

* Rest for 20 seconds between each set of all four exercises.

Take a 1-minute rest before beginning push-up and ab routine below.

5. Handstand push-ups	5	5
6. Diamond push-ups	5	30
7. Sit-ups	10	25
8. Crunches	10	50
9. Leg lifts	10	10

* Rest for 30 seconds between each set of the 5 exercises.

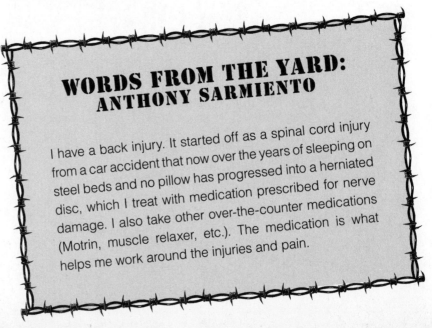

WORDS FROM THE YARD:
ANTHONY SARMIENTO

I have a back injury. It started off as a spinal cord injury from a car accident that now over the years of sleeping on steel beds and no pillow has progressed into a herniated disc, which I treat with medication prescribed for nerve damage. I also take other over-the-counter medications (Motrin, muscle relaxer, etc.). The medication is what helps me work around the injuries and pain.

CHAPTER 15

Israel Alberto Guillén [J-30121]

Inmate Rap Sheet

Name: Israel Guillén	**CDCR#:** J-30121
Age: 39	**Height:** 6'0"
Weight before prison: 215 pounds	
Weight after beginning prison workout plan: 215 pounds	
Length of incarceration: Life	
Time served: 19 years	

About the Inmate: Israel mainly works out for self-defense, and he's very intense about his routine. He keeps that intensity going staying off any body part that is giving him pain. Israel admits his endurance has greatly improved with the workouts he currently does in prison.

Stretching

While we believe stretching is best after a workout and that a warm-up should last between 5 and 10 minutes, Israel stretches *before* his routine. He holds each stretch for thirty seconds on each side. While we question the benefit of this technique as compared with post-workout stretching, the inmates who take this approach do the following stretches:

1. Wide-stance toe reach
2. Wide-stance torso stretch with one arm up
3. Wide-stance ground touch (bent over at waist)
4. Close-stance toe touch (head touching knee caps)
5. Standing knee hold (pulling knee in toward chest)
6. Standing quad stretch (pulling heel back toward buttocks)

Again, there's nothing wrong with brief stretching before a workout to loosen up, but we do recommend that you stretch after the following routine as well.

DAY 1

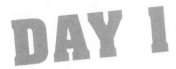

Israel's day 1 routine is a great upper-body circuit. The sequence of exercises is very well thought out—Israel starts with a multijoint movement that uses the back before going to a single-joint movement that uses the biceps (muscles that assist in all back exercises). He then switches to multijoint movements that incorporate the chest and finishes with a triceps exercise (a muscle that assists in chest exercises).

But before you do any of this, Israel recommends that you start this first day out with a one-mile run. Start out the first quarter mile slow, then pick up the pace to a little less than half speed at the middle half mile. Then finish up the last quarter mile at a little quicker than half speed. This increase in speed is a gradual warm up and will help you avoid injury. If you were to start running at a quick pace you risk pulling muscles or tearing ligaments and/or tendons because your body simply isn't ready to perform at high level before warming up.

Upper Body
(Back, Chest, Biceps, and Triceps)

EXERCISE	SETS	REPS
1a. Regular pull-ups	5	5
1b. Biceps curls	5	10–20
1c. Incline push-ups	5	15
1d. Bar dips	5	10

* Do 5 circuits of the above with 4–6 seconds of rest between each.

EXERCISE	SETS	REPS
2a. Behind-the-head pull-ups	5	5
2b. Biceps curls	5	10–20
2c. Incline push-ups	5	15
2d. Dips	5	10

* Do 5 circuits of the above with 4–6 seconds of rest between each.

DAY 2

After today's routine be sure to stretch your quads and hamstrings with the quad stretch and standing toe touch. This day 2 routine has a lot of leg exercises, so you'll need to stretch afterward to avoid muscle tightening. But before you get going, start today with a 1-mile run done in the same fashion as day 1.

Legs

EXERCISE	SETS	REPS
1. Alternating forward lunges	1	100 (each leg)
2. Calf raises	1	200
3. Alternating reverse lunges	1	100 (each leg)
4. Calf raises	1	200
5. Hanging oblique leg raise	5	5
6. Crunches	5	30

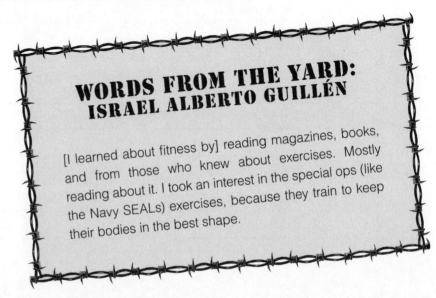

WORDS FROM THE YARD: ISRAEL ALBERTO GUILLÉN

[I learned about fitness by] reading magazines, books, and from those who knew about exercises. Mostly reading about it. I took an interest in the special ops (like the Navy SEALs) exercises, because they train to keep their bodies in the best shape.

DAY 3

Don't be fooled by this day 3 workout because it has only two exercises. It contains 200 burpies with 200 built-in push-ups along with 100 pull-ups. Start things off with a 1-mile run done in the same fashion as day 1.

Back and Chest

EXERCISE	SETS	REPS
1a. Palm-in, palm-out pull-ups	20	5
1b. 6-count burpies	20	10

* 20 supersets are done with just 10 seconds of rest between sets.

DAY 4

Israel mixes up his workout on day 4 by recommending that you do 100 side busters to kick things off. Do these after stretching but before the daily 1-mile run done in the same style as described on day 1. Once you've completed the run, take a 3-minute rest before starting the following exercises.

Legs

EXERCISE	SETS	REPS
1. Step-ups knee-crunch	1	100 (each side)

* Take a 2-minute rest after step-ups.

EXERCISE	SETS	REPS
2. Calf raises	1	200
3. Squats	1	100
4. Calf raises	1	200
5. Squats	1	100

DAY 5

Start today off with the 1-mile run in the style described on day 1.

Chest, Triceps, Abs, and Forearms

EXERCISE	SETS	REPS
1a. Decline push-ups	20	20
1b. Back arm presses	20	10
1c. Hanging oblique leg raises	20	25
1d. Reverse curls	20	20

* 20 circuits of the 4 exercises done with 20 seconds of rest between sets.

WORDS FROM THE YARD: ISRAEL ALBERTO GUILLÉN

Due to my exhaustive exercises, I feel like a linebacker! I feel powerful! I'm 215 pounds and thirty-six years old, so I'm surprised that my health, flexibility, and energy is as good as it is. Being my age, I'm now focusing on my abs, legs, chest, and arms, but I train myself to be in good condition. I do a lot of shadow boxing because it keeps me tight and lets me know how fast or slow I can go if I need to defend myself. Shadow boxing and front kicks are great warm ups! Sometimes I'll do 10 sets of 100 punches, 15 push-ups, 15 front kicks (each leg), and 15 jump squats. I'll do my 10-minute ab workout before and after this exercise and believe me, you'll get a great sweat and it will make you feel like a champ!

CHAPTER 16

Shant Der Boghossian [H-17796]

Inmate Rap Sheet

Name: Shant Der Boghossian	**CDCR#:** H-17796
Age: 42	**Height:** 5'10"
Weight before prison: Unknown	
Weight after beginning prison workout plan: Unknown	
Length of incarceration: Unknown	
Time served: Unknown	

About the Inmate: As you look at this section of workouts you'll notice that Shant's routines are clear and well organized. He manages his time well by spreading his routine out during the day; he always starts his routine by doing abdominal exercises before breakfast. He then performs his strength/resistance training early in the day before completing an aerobic workout later in the afternoon/early evening.

You will likely notice that the workouts provided by Shant (the model in the gray shorts in the pictures earlier in the book) don't contain any pull-ups or dips. Why? Because these routines come from inmates who work out while in a Security Housing Unit (SHU, pronounced "shoe") during Administrative Segregation (AD-SEG), which is similar to solitary confinement. For their own safety and the safety of others, many inmates are kept separate from all other inmates for a predetermined amount of time in order to keep gang-related violence and other incidents to a minimum. While placed in the SHU/AD-SEG, inmates do not have access to pull-up bars or dip bars, but fellow inmates can easily tell when another inmate is released from the SHU—he's always shredded.

However, if you try Shant's workout and want to add pull-ups and dips to the routine, feel free.

DAY 1

6:00 A.M.—Stomach

EXERCISE	SETS	REPS
1. Cross-leg sit-ups (left/right)	5	15
2. Oblique crunches (left/right)	5	15
3. Leg lifts	5	30
4. Crunches	5	30

Note: One set of regular push-ups to failure will determine the number of repetitions performed during later sets of regular push-ups, wide push-ups, and diamond push-ups. For example: If you perform 100 push-ups to failure ("x"), you will do 50 push-ups in some sets and 33 in others (½x and ⅓x respectively).

8:00 A.M.—Chest/Triceps

EXERCISE	SETS	REPS
1. Regular push-ups	1	To failure (x)
2. Regular push-ups	10	½x
3. Wide push-ups (hands pointed out)	10	⅓x
4. Diamond push-ups	10	⅓x
5. Double-handed kick-outs	7	20
6. Single-handed kick-outs	7	10
7. Palms-down back arm press	7	20
8. Palms-in back arm press	7	20

3:00 P.M.—Cardio

EXERCISE	SETS	REPS
1. Burpies	1	100–300

DAY 2

6:00 A.M.—Stomach

EXERCISE	SETS	REPS
1. Cross-leg sit-ups (left/right)	5	15
2. Oblique crunches (left/right)	5	15
3. Leg lifts	5	30
4. Crunches	5	30

8:00 A.M.—Calisthenics

EXERCISE	SETS	REPS
1. Jumping jacks	1	100
2. 6-count burpies	1	20
3. Squats	1	50
4. 3-count chain breakers	1	50
5. 8-count burpies	1	20
6. Lunges	1	50
7. Belly busters	1	50
8. 10-count burpies	1	20
9. Butterflies	1	50
10. Navy SEAL burpies	1	20
11. Calf raises	1	150
12. Arm rotations	1	300
13. 6-count burpies	1	20
14. Squats	1	50
15. Windmills	1	50
16. 8-count burpies	1	20
17. Lunges	1	50
18. Cherry pickers	1	50
19. 10-count burpies	1	20
20. Jumping jacks	1	100

3:00 P.M.—Cardio

EXERCISE	SETS	REPS
1. Burpies (your choice)	1	100–300

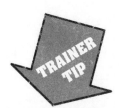

TRAINER TIP

Use the time you save by not driving to the gym to increase the length of your workout. That way you'll see results faster and occupy more time not reserved for eating.

DAY 3

* "21s" are a series of three ranges of motion (7 repetitions for each range) while doing curls. The first range is from the base of a curl to where the elbow reaches a 90-degree angle (the first half of a full curl). The second range starts with the elbow at a 90-degree angle and goes up to the chest (the second half of a full curl). The third range of motion is actually a full curl, just as you would perform it in other routines. "21s" are a great way to develop the biceps and improve strength through the "sticking point," where the exercise is biomechanically most challenging; at 90 degrees of elbow flexion.

6:00 A.M.—Stomach

EXERCISE	SETS	REPS
1. Cross-leg sit-ups (left/right)	5	15
2. Oblique crunches (left/right)	5	15
3. Leg lifts	5	30
4. Crunches	5	30

8:00 A.M.—Biceps/Shoulders/Forearms

EXERCISE	SETS	REPS
1. Curls	7	20
2. Reverse-grip curls	7	20
3. Single-arm curls	7	10
4. Hammer curls	7	20
5. 21s*	5	21
6. Bent-over row	7	30
7. Upright row	7	20
8. Double-hand front raise	7	10
9. Lawn mowers	7	15
10. Front shrugs	10	30
11. Behind back shrugs	10	30
12. Wrist curls	10	25
13. Reverse wrist curls	10	25

3:00 P.M.—Cardio

EXERCISE	SETS	REPS
1. Burpies (your choice)	1	100–300

DAY 4

6:00 A.M.—Stomach

EXERCISE	SETS	REPS
1. Cross-leg sit-ups (left/right)	5	15
2. Oblique crunches (left/right)	5	15
3. Leg lifts	5	30
4. Crunches	5	30

8:00 A.M. "Rodeo" of Burpies

EXERCISE	SETS	REPS
1. Navy SEAL burpies	1	100
2. 10-count burpies	7	100
3. 8-count burpies	7	100
4. 6-count burpies	7	100

3:00 P.M.—Cardio

EXERCISE	SETS	REPS
1. Burpies (your choice)	1	100–300

DAY 5

6:00 A.M.—Stomach

EXERCISE	SETS	REPS
1. Cross-leg sit-ups (left/right)	5	15
2. Oblique crunches (left/right)	5	15
3. Leg lifts	5	30
4. Crunches	5	30

8:00 A.M.—Legs and Lower Back

EXERCISE	SETS	REPS
1. Squats	10	20–30
2. Lunges (each leg)	10	15–20
3. Single-leg squats (each leg)	7	15–20
4. Bulgarian squats (each leg)	7	15–20
5. Double-leg calf raises	5	50
6. Single-leg calf raises	5	30
7. Good mornings	10	15
8. Windmills (with weight)	10	15

3:00 P.M.—Cardio

EXERCISE	SETS	REPS
1. Burpies (your choice)	1	100–300

DAY 6

6:00 A.M.—Stomach

EXERCISE	SETS	REPS
1. Cross-leg sit-ups (left/right)	5	15
2. Oblique crunches (left/right)	5	15
3. Leg lifts	5	30
4. Crunches	5	30

8:00 A.M.—Calisthenics

EXERCISE	SETS	REPS
1. Jumping jacks	1	50
2. Push-ups	1	20
3. Navy SEAL burpies	1	20
4. Squats	1	30
5. 3-count chain breakers	1	30
6. Push-ups	1	20
7. Navy SEAL burpies	1	20
8. Lunges	1	30
9. Belly busters	1	30
10. Push-ups	1	20
11. Navy SEAL burpies	1	20
12. Butterflies	1	30
13. Push-ups	1	20
14. Navy SEAL burpies	1	20
15. Calf raises (each leg)	1	100
16. Arm rotations	1	300
17. Push-ups	1	20
18. Navy SEAL burpies	1	20
19. Jumping jacks	1	50

3:00 P.M.—Cardio

EXERCISE	SETS	REPS
1. Burpies (your choice)	1	100–300

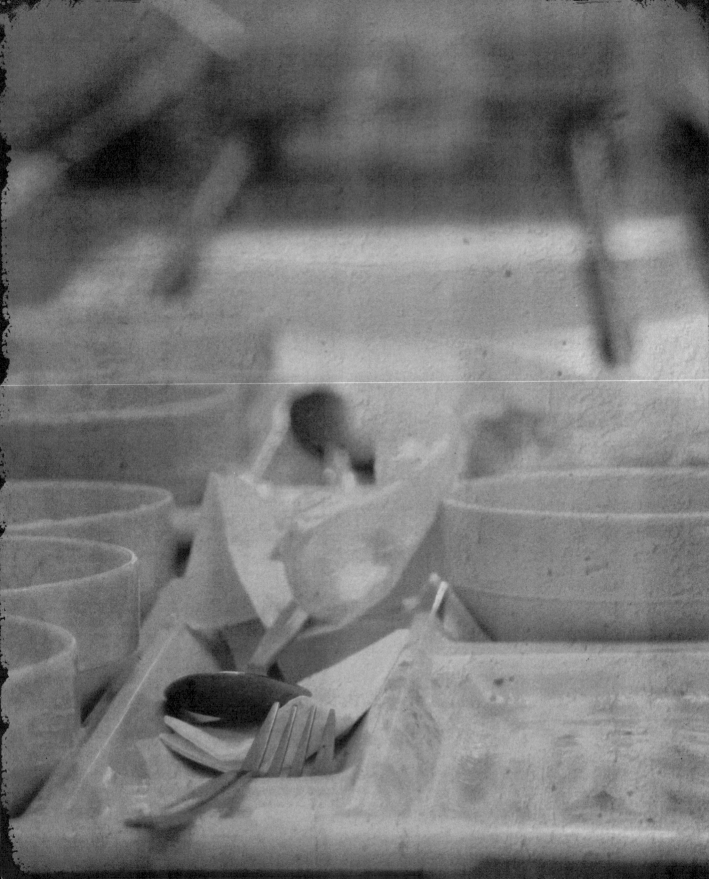

PART 5
Diet

A prison diet is notoriously bad. Yes, things have come a long way since inmates were only given bread and water, but correctional facilities still give poor-quality food to inmates. In addition, even the foods inmates can buy at the prison commissary or the foods that can be included in care packages from family and friends (go to *www.californiaqp.com* to see what can be sent inside) are highly processed, sugar-laden, or just plain junk: cheese puffs, cookies, popcorn, pastas, chips, pastries, candy, and crackers of all varieties are available.

Unfortunately loved ones can't send leafy green vegetables, fresh fruit, or lean meat like you would find at a grocery store. But, regardless of the quality of the food they are served, the inmates who exercise consistently are healthy, amazingly fit, lean, and strong. Why? Because they have educated themselves on the subject of nutrition and refuse to negate the hard work they put into their workouts/bodies. In fact, most inmates ask for items that aren't edible: socks, toothpaste, deodorant, coffee, headphones, sneakers, hats, vitamins, body wash, pencil sharpeners, pens, shorts, bar soap, toothbrushes, and laundry detergent. These inmates do whatever it takes to remain healthy, strong, and alive, and they avoid eating anything that will throw them off track. If you want to remain—or become—healthy, you must do the same. Read on to learn how.

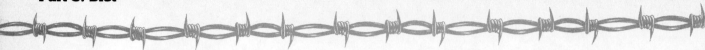

Play by the Rules

If you want to follow a healthy diet and lose weight safely there are some basic rules—outlined below—that you can follow to get started. Fortunately, you have more freedom when it comes to when and what you eat than our inmates, but just like them, you need to take responsibility for your own diet and your own health. Use the following diet rules to keep you on the straight and narrow.

1. **Eat less:** If you are overweight, it is likely that you overeat. Today's portion sizes tend to be much larger than the serving size you should actually eat. For example, consider the amount of pasta you're likely served at popular Italian restaurants. Those portions are often four, five, or six times more food and calories than you actually need. Try inverting the ratio of what you might see on your plate at these restaurants (four times more vegetables and one-fourth of the pasta) and you'll have a much healthier and a more satisfying meal.

2. **Burn more calories than you take in:** Don't you dare think that you can eat more now that you're exercising—especially if you're overweight. If you want to slim down you need to burn more calories than you're eating. It's only when you create a caloric deficit that you will begin to lose weight.

3. **Eat a balanced diet:** All food is made up of three macronutrients: carbohydrates, proteins, and fats. You need all three for energy (carbs and fat) and tissue repair (protein), so don't eliminate any of them. The food plate outlined by the USDA at *www.choosemyplate.gov* will give you a good idea as to how much of each nutrient you should consume. Also check out *www.eatnakednow.com*, which is run by Nutritional Therapy Practitioner Margaret Floyd. Floyd's site outlines practical ways to improve your diet by cooking healthy meals with whole foods, choosing healthier products, and making small changes in what you eat that can make big changes in how you feel.

4. **Cut out sweets:** Most sweets contain high-fructose corn syrup— avoid it as much as you can. Ingesting too much HFCS brings the

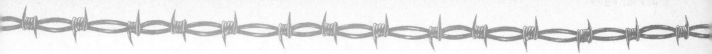

risk of liver damage, increased LDL cholesterol levels (the bad kind), increased risk of weight gain, and an increased risk of diabetes.

5. **Pour sugar-saturated drinks down the drain:** Cutting out sugary beverages is an easy way to cut out unnecessary calories. Juices, sodas, alcohol, and energy drinks all have calories you simply don't need.

6. **Cut out fried foods:** The oil in which most foods are fried contains unhealthy trans fats. Fried food also has a ton of calories and often doesn't contain the vitamins and minerals needed to maintain and improve health.

7. **Eat more leafy green and multicolored vegetables:** Veggies, especially colorful ones, are high in vitamins and minerals, fill you up faster because of their high water content, have very few calories, and help food move through the digestive tract because they are high in fiber.

8. **Eat more fruit:** Like vegetables, fruits are also high in vitamins and minerals. However, they have more calories because of their naturally occurring sugar so don't go overboard.

9. **Stay away from starchy foods like pasta and bread:** These foods aren't bad for you, but you don't want to eat too much because they add a lot of calories, don't fill you up, and can cause a spike in blood sugar and insulin levels—all of which can easily make you gain weight.

Following these basic tips will get you on the right track to healthy eating, however please realize that if you have special dietary needs due to allergies, a vegetarian/vegan diet, or chronic disorders, you should visit a nutritionist to make sure the plan you're choosing is the best—and the safest—plan for you. Nutritionists can really help you refine your diet without eliminating all the pleasure you may take from food, and their qualifications and level of expertise on diet greatly exceed ours, so take advantage of them.

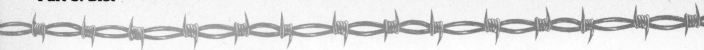

Felon FAQs

At the beginning of every year nearly every TV talk show in the United States begins broadcasting reports on how to shed extra pounds. This is also when trainers start to hear the following questions from all corners of the gym:

"Should I supplement?"

"Is sugar bad for me?"

"How many calories should I take in each day?"

"I've heard I should graze throughout the day and eat small meals. Is that true?"

But whether you're looking to drop some pounds as part of a New Year's resolution or are just looking to shape up, the answers to the above questions are simple and haven't changed: You shouldn't have to. No. It depends on your desired weight and activity level. Yes. We go into greater detail below, but we can't do your homework for you. This book contains great workouts to get you in shape, but you are accountable for your own well-being and need to research what it means to eat right. We'll give you a few places to start, but all-in-all it is in your hands.

 I've heard it's good to eat a lot of protein, but no carbs or fats. Is that true?

No. Fruits and vegetables are carbohydrates. Don't be afraid of them. Not only are vegetables great sources of vitamins and minerals but they also have wonderful amounts of fiber to aid in digestion and elimination. Half of your diet should come from vegetables. Eat up. They are also extremely low in calories so don't fret that eating a lot of lettuce, cabbage, spinach, kale, celery, and other leafy greens will pack on the pounds. What you need to avoid is too much of the starchy, complex carbohydrates (bread, pasta, grain) that cause a spike in blood sugar levels and trigger the release of insulin, which can easily lead to weight gain. A little of these types of carbohydrates is fine, just don't overdo it by eating too much. A good way to think about it is that more pasta or grain than what can fit in the palm of your hand (one-quarter to a half cup) is too much. If you look at your dinner plate, roughly one-eighth of your meal should come from starchy carbs.

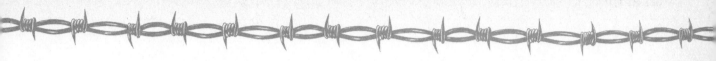

Fat

Fat is another misunderstood nutrient. It is a concentrated form/source of energy that, at nine calories per gram, has just over twice as many calories per gram as carbohydrate and protein, which each have four calories per gram. Fats come in two categories, saturated and unsaturated.

Saturated fats are solid at room temperature. They often come from red meat, poultry, pork, and dairy products. Eat these foods in moderation to reduce your intake of saturated fat. Studies prove the correlation between heart disease and diets high in saturated fat time and time again. Check out the American Heart Association website (*www.heart.org*) to learn more.

Unsaturated fats are liquid at room temperature. They come from plant oils (sesame, olive, safflower, avocados) and nuts (almonds, walnuts, peanuts, etc.). The great thing about these fats is their ability to get rid of newly formed cholesterol in your arterial walls. Eat unsaturated fats in place of saturated fats but remember to moderate. Too many calories from unsaturated fat can still lead to weight gain. Be careful. About one-eighth of your plate should be a source of unsaturated fat.

Protein

Protein, which should be a part of any meal or snack that you eat, has many functions, but for the sake of exercise and fitness its main job is to build and repair body tissues. The tricky thing about protein is that it usually comes attached to fat.

Meat is a great source of protein, but literally you'll have to trim the fat (in solid form easily visible to your naked eye) off your steak or chicken breast in order to keep saturated fats to a minimum. Nuts have both fat (in their natural oils) and protein. Beans are an even better source of protein. They have fiber and a lot of water, both of which will make you feel full and prevent overeating. So feel free to eat these protein-filled foods—just keep your eating in check.

Q *Should I take supplements?*

A You shouldn't have to supplement in order to maintain a healthy weight, but if you're looking to add muscle mass, a well-made protein powder

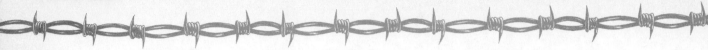

is a good idea. For those basic supplements we suggest taking a look at Body360 Nutritionals at *www.body360nutritionals.com*. Their founder and CEO is a well-educated and experienced trainer who sees dozens of sub-standard products on the market and strives to offer the highest-quality formulations. In addition, multivitamins are a good idea to make sure you get enough of the important vitamins and minerals that might be absent in your diet.

Is sugar bad for me?

No. Natural sugars found in fruit and vegetables are not bad for you. But processed sugar, specifically high-fructose corn syrup, is bad for the reasons discussed earlier on in this part. In order to avoid HFCS you have to read the labels of what you're buying at the grocery store. If you see "high-fructose corn syrup" put it back on the shelf and look for another item without this ingredient.

How many calories should I take in each day?

The number of calories your body needs to maintain a specific weight is known as your basal metabolic rate (BMR). That number depends on your age, sex, height, level of activity, and desired weight. Women need fewer calories than men, since males have more muscle, which burns more calories. Tall people need more calories because their bodies are naturally larger and need more fuel. Older people need fewer calories because their metabolic systems have been slowing down year after year. People who exercise need more calories because they burn more. The variables are endless! Check out *www.bmi-calculator.net/bmr-calculator/* to learn your estimated caloric need.

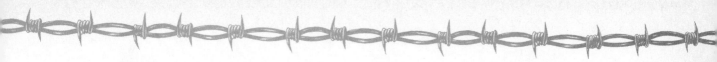

Q *I've heard I should graze throughout the day and eat small meals. Is that true?*

 This question relates to what we've covered about eating fewer starchy carbs, avoiding processed sugars, and keeping your blood-sugar and insulin levels steady to avoid gaining weight. It is a myth that eating throughout the day speeds up your metabolism, but eating small meals (five or six per day) helps to curb cravings and prevent overeating during regular meal times.

It's important for you to keep in mind that snacks are, in fact, small meals. Do you crave a nibble between lunch and dinner? Don't resist that urge. Have a small snack with some protein, fat, and carbohydrates (fruit with nuts is a great example) and you've started a great habit.

AFTERWORD

Out of the California Clink

Probation (prō-BĀ-shən)

1. subjection of an individual to a period of testing and trial to ascertain fitness

2. the action of suspending the sentence of a convicted offender and giving the offender freedom during good behavior under the supervision of a probation officer (*Merriam Webster's Collegiate Dictionary*, 11th edition)

Probation: No word could be as fitting for the journey you have undertaken. You've decided to put yourself through a period of testing to see if you have what it takes to get fit outside the walls of both a prison and a gym. Think of this undertaking as a virtual release.

You now have the tools to exercise wherever your imagination takes you. You're not bound by workout equipment. Instead you're practicing back-to-basics fitness and using your body—the most intricate, well-designed, and fascinating machine in the world—as it is meant to be used. Who would have thought the user's manual for such a complex machine would come down from West Coast prisons?

The training programs sent to us by inmates of the California State Prison system show no mercy to any muscle group. Your chest, back, legs, shoulders, forearms, biceps, triceps, and abdominals will definitely be sore after you complete one of these workouts. However, once you see your body begin to respond to these routines all the pain and hard work will be worth it. You will begin to see definition in your body that you haven't seen in years. You will be the envy of your coworkers. Doctors will praise you. Friends will pester you to share your secret. Family members will pretend they are not jealous that you have unlocked your inner inmate. Share your routines with them the same way the inmates shared them with you. Work hard. And congratulations on becoming felon fit.

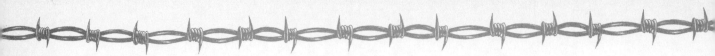

Index

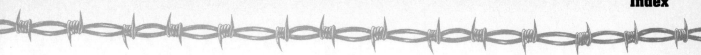

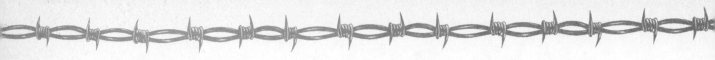

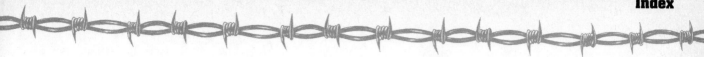

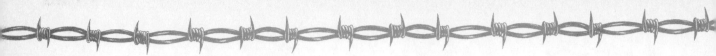

R

S

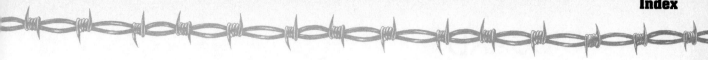

About the Authors

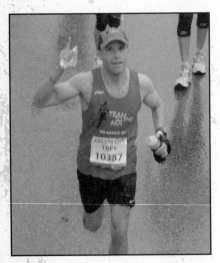

Trey Teufel is a certified personal trainer (NASM), a graduate of Indiana University (Bloomington), and a lover of Cleveland Indians baseball, marathon training, and all things fitness-related. He has been a personal trainer for nearly a decade in the demanding cities of New York and Los Angeles. Trey currently resides in Los Angeles around the corner from Bill.

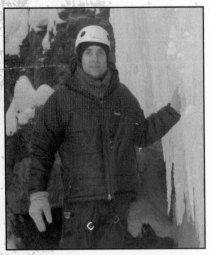

William "Bill" Kroger is a criminal attorney in Los Angeles. In his twelve years of practice he has visited dozens of jails and prisons throughout the United States. When visiting his clients in prison he noticed they were always in great shape and when he saw them upon their release he was amazed at how fit they had become. Being an avid rock and ice climber and an expert skier, Bill was used to working out on a regular basis with weights and machines, but found the prison workouts to be extremely challenging and fun. At age fifty, Bill is a dedicated husband, father, and courtroom warrior, and is in the best shape of his life.